gratitude♡cleanse

21 DAYS TO CLEANSE YOUR BODY, OPEN YOUR MIND, AND AWAKEN YOUR HEART

GEMMA FARRELL

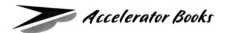

Accelerator Books

Published by Accelerator Books

For information, please contact Accelerator Books, P.O. Box 1241, Princeton, NJ 08542.

Designed by Eve Siegel Designs
Typeset by Rainbow Graphics

ISBN: 978-0-984966-0-8

Dedicated to the Gratitude Yoga students—they are my finest teachers—and to my best friend, Jack, and my five other best friends, our children, Marian, Emmanuelle, Richard, Jack, and Tade—they are gifts beyond measure, every one.

Acknowledgments

The contents of this book have been inspired by and derived from various sources, most notably from the writings of Thich Nhat Hanh, Sarah Powers, Natalia Rose, and Lama Willa Miller.

Many of the recipes herein come from the wonderful NYC restaurant Pure Food and Wine and its founders, Sarma Melngailis and Matthew Kenny, as well as from Natalia Rose, whose work in the raw-food community has been invaluable. I also have been enlightened and educated by the amazing healer Gil Jacobs. I am indebted to these teachers and to countless others who go unnamed here. May their light reach you.

I have to express my gratitude to my husband and best friend, Jack, whose abiding love sustains me. I am immensely thankful for my children, Marian, Emmanuelle, Richard, Jack, and Tade, who show me the meaning of compassion and unconditional love each and every day.

Contents

Introduction

Health is a state of complete harmony of the body, mind, and spirit. When one is free from physical disabilities and mental distractions, the gates of the soul open.

—B. K. S. Iyengar

Welcome to the start of your Gratitude Cleanse. It is wonderful that you have decided to take this journey toward wholeness. This Body, Mind, Spirit Cleanse is designed to span three full weeks. It incorporates philosophical and spiritual reflection, yoga, meditation, breathing exercises, and other lifestyle changes, as well as some work with your diet, to promote cleansing and healing on the physical and emotional fronts.

The nutritional component of the cleanse relies primarily on the power of raw foods—fresh fruits and vegetables and their juices—to detoxify and energize your system at a cellular level. I encourage you to think of the cleanse as an *indulgence* rather than a program of deprivation. You will be enjoying unlimited amounts of raw food—vibrant, juicy fruits and crunchy, flavorful vegetables—flooding your body with pure, fresh ingredients in their natural, unprocessed state. Consuming unlimited amounts of raw foods simply crowds out the less helpful foods so that the fruits and vegetables can do their cleansing and revitalizing work.

An important feature of this three-week cleanse is spending at least one full week eating only raw fruits and vegetables and using plenty of fresh fruit and vegetable juices and smoothies to remove accumulated toxins and provide the benefits of vibrant vitamin-, mineral-, and enzyme-rich raw foods.

I suggest that you make the transition to a completely raw diet of fruits and vegetables in the following way:

Week 1: Eliminate all refined sugar and white flour. This means no bread, pasta, cakes, cookies, pastries, and so on.
Week 2: Also eliminate animal products, including meat, poultry, fish, eggs, and dairy (i.e., milk, butter, cheese, and yogurt).
Week 3: Also eliminate all cooked and/or processed foods and eat only raw fruits and vegetables for this entire week.

Of course, if you prefer to progress at a different pace than the one just outlined, you are welcome to slow down or accelerate the process at any point. You may tailor the cleanse to fit your needs and interests, and I invite you to find the appropriate balance for you.

Throughout the entire three-week cleanse, please try to adhere to the following guidelines:

❖ Drink as much pure water as possible, at least ten 8-ounce glasses each day.

❖ Begin each day by drinking a cup of hot water with lemon juice, and drink several glasses of plain water during the day.

❖ Drink at least one 12-ounce glass of freshly juiced green lemonade each day on an empty stomach, ideally around 11 a.m. Gradually work your way up to 20 to 40 ounces each day.

Green Lemonade

1 head romaine lettuce or celery

5-6 stalks kale (preferably lacinato, or "elephant," kale)

1 whole lemon

1-3 apples (I recommend Granny Smith or Fuji)—optional, as needed for sweetness

1-2 inches fresh ginger—optional

Please use organic produce for this recipe.

❖ Limit your eating to the daylight hours—try not to eat after the sun goes down. Eat only fresh fruit until noon each day (no other food prior to 12 noon). Always eat fruit by itself, separate from other foods.

❖ Soak raw nuts and seeds in water for several hours or overnight to make them easier to digest. Eating nuts and seeds will slow down the cleansing process, so please use them wisely.

❖ Use dry brushing to release toxins through the skin and stimulate the lymphatic system. Detailed instructions appear in Day Fourteen.

In addition to working with food to cleanse your body, you also may want to take these three weeks to incorporate other lifestyle habits that will promote well-being and a sense of inner peace. I invite you to make it a priority over the coming weeks to

rest—Get plenty of sleep so that your body can rejuvenate itself.

breathe—Practice simple breathing techniques throughout the day in your car, at work, while preparing dinner. Information about specific breathing techniques appears in Day Six.

sweat—Our skin is our largest organ of elimination. Allow your pores to open and release toxins. Yoga class is often a good place to sweat. You also may undertake a different form of exercise, use a sauna or steam room, or simply take a hot bath each day using Epsom salts or mustard powder to induce your pores to open.

go outdoors—Take in sunlight and fresh air for at least ten minutes each day. Make every effort to build this into your daily routine by taking a walk, a run, a swim, or a bike ride, doing some gardening, or just spending time outside with a friend or a favorite book.

move and stretch—Practice some yoga, either at home or in yoga class, every day, even if it is only for a few minutes first thing in the morning or before going to sleep. This book provides instructions for a different yoga pose for each day of the cleanse, which will give you the chance to spend a few minutes exploring yoga on your own each day. If you can commit to attending more yoga classes during these three weeks, it will be of great benefit. You also may want to vary your exercise routine a bit, perhaps including Pilates, dance, running, swimming, tennis, golf, or other physical activities that you enjoy.

meditate—Commit to meditate for at least five minutes each day. You will find instructions on the basic meditation technique, The Three Arrivals, in Day One.

unplug—Eliminate distractions so that you can cultivate mindfulness throughout your day. Limit your computer and cell phone usage, and resist watching TV, listening to empty music, or seeing mindless movies. So much of our precious time is squandered on mind-numbing media.

get inspired—Read enlightening books, and listen to at least a few minutes of classical music each day. You may want to set your car and/or home radio to a classical music station and leave it there for these three weeks.

and above all . . .

cultivate gratitude—Dwell on the people and circumstances in your life for which you are thankful. Our lives are replete with blessings. We need to remind ourselves of how truly fortunate we are. Allow the transforming power of gratitude to awaken your heart.

be present—As often as possible throughout these twenty-one days, bring yourself into the present moment and reside there, free from preoccupations about the past or the future. Give yourself and the people in your life the gift of your genuine presence.

HOW TO USE THIS BOOK

> I think to myself that this day is a day to live fully, and I make the vow to live each moment of it in a way that is beautiful, solid, and free.
>
> —*Thich Nhat Hanh*

There is much to say about cleansing, nutrition, yoga, meditation, and wisdom practices. This book only skims the surface. It is meant to be a practical guide to transforming your lifestyle and the way in which you relate to yourself and others. To that end, the book is organized on a day-by-day basis. Each daily chapter contains the following components:

—A *quote* for the day, along with some information about a philosophical or spiritual theme for that day, and meditation, breath work, yoga, and wisdom practices to cultivate qualities such as mindfulness, compassion, generosity, gratitude, and patience.

—A wisdom-related *exercise of the day* that invites reflection and encourages you to develop a deeper understanding of yourself and the world.

—A *yoga pose of the day*. If you enjoy practicing yoga, the yoga pose of the day provides you with an opportunity to explore some of the basic, foundational yoga poses, or *asanas*. I suggest that you carve out some regular time, perhaps either first thing in morning or just before going to sleep, to practice the pose of the day for a few minutes.

—Some information about *nutrition and cleansing*.

—A selection of *recipes* for the day. Several recipes are included for each day so that you can try them out as you move along through the cleanse. All the daily recipes are also included in a broader listing of recipes that comprises the final chapter of this book.

GETTING READY

Following is a preliminary shopping list for the cleanse. It is by no means comprehensive and is intended merely to give you a starting point. As you move through the next three weeks, you likely will add or eliminate items as you discover what appeals to you. Day Seventeen contains more detailed information about some of the food items listed below that might be new to you.

Gratitude Cleanse Shopping List

water (If you do not have a water filter or distiller, you will want to purchase plenty of spring or distilled water.)

lots of fresh fruit, especially
pineapple
melon
berries
grapes
apples
lemons

any raw vegetables you like, such as
spinach
tomatoes
avocados
carrots
broccoli
zucchini

also be sure to include, for your daily green lemonade
celery
romaine lettuce
lacinato kale
lemons
fresh ginger

raw nuts and seeds, including
almonds
walnuts
macadamia nuts
sunflower seeds
pumpkin seeds (pepitas)
sesame seeds
hemp seeds
pine nuts
(avoid peanuts)

raw nut butters, such as
raw almond butter
raw cashew butter
raw sunflower butter
raw sesame seed butter (tahini)

cold-pressed oils, such as
flax seed oil
extra-virgin cold-pressed olive oil
sesame oil
coconut oil

miscellaneous seasonings/condiments, such as
raw honey
raw agave syrup
stevia (I prefer liquid stevia from NuStevia Naturals.)
Nama Shoyu soy sauce
Celtic sea salt
powdered seaweed seasoning such as kelp or dulse
nutritional yeast
cayenne pepper

Equipment/Detox Supplies

natural bristle skin brush for dry brushing—These natural bristle brushes are used to slough off skin cells and stimulate circulation and lymphatic flow. Many of the body brushes are too stiff. I like the Bass brand best. Please see more information and instructions on dry brushing in Day Fourteen.

tongue scraper—The metal tongue scrapers are far better than the plastic ones. I like the Dr. Tung brand.

neti pot—A neti pot is a small vessel, usually made of ceramic or metal, used for irrigating the nasal passages, a practice that began as an ancient ayurvedic technique. It has become widely accepted as a home remedy to relieve such conditions as allergies, colds, and mild sinus infections. Nasal irrigation can be helpful during a cleanse because the detoxification process often produces excess mucus. More detailed information about use of a neti pot appears in Day Twelve.

essential oils for aromatherapy—I recommend Aura Cacia or Windmere brand essential oils. Myriad essential oils are available, each with its own properties and benefits. Day Seven offers a brief listing of commonly used essential oils and their uses and benefits.

juicer—If you do not already own a juicer, I strongly suggest that you consider borrowing or buying one for this cleanse. Fresh raw fruit and vegetable juices are powerful cleansing agents and absolutely essential to a successful raw cleansing diet. There are many juicers on the market. My recommendation is to find one with a wide opening that is quick and easy to use and clean. This will ensure that juicing does not become a time-consuming, labor-intensive process. I prefer the Breville juicer for its price point (in the $100–$200 range) and the fact that it has a large mouth and is quick and easy to both use and clean. However, its less powerful motor leaves much of the vital juice in the pulp. Green Life and Omega ($300–$600) are excellent brands if you have room in your budget for a more expensive juicer.

blender—While a basic blender will do just fine for the purposes of this cleanse, the higher-quality blenders such as the Vitamix or the K-Tec are well worth the higher price (around $400) if you decide to make raw soups, smoothies, nut milks, and desserts a regular part of your diet beyond the three-week cleanse.

THE DAY BEFORE

> All beings have the seed of purity within that may be transformed and fully developed into wisdom and compassion.
> —*Translation of the well-known Buddhist mantra:*
> *Om Mani Padme Hum*

Our minds can be seen as soil containing many "seeds" or potentialities—seeds of joy and compassion and understanding, as well as seeds of aggression, violence, and selfishness. What we cultivate and nurture in our hearts and minds is what will flourish for us in our lives.

It is encouraging to know that we possess the potential for growth in many different directions. As you adopt some of the diet and lifestyle changes recommended in this cleanse, it may be helpful to recall this concept of *seed potential*. Recognizing and touching the positive seeds within ourselves and others is the first step in promoting positive change and in growing a compassionate, expansive, and wise heart.

Remember that the dietary focus of this cleanse is on including lots of fresh fruit and vegetables—as much as you can eat—rather than on depriving yourself.

Bear in mind that raw foods are potent agents for change—they stir things up. This is why you will want to transition somewhat gradually, taking several weeks to eliminate refined sugar and flour, animal products, and cooked foods and adding more and more raw food as the cleanse progresses.

> . . . the life force energy (of raw food) is very powerful and can help the body heal itself. The live enzymes within raw foods serve as catalysts to support every human function. Because your store of enzymes runs dangerously low in adulthood, a

sudden influx of live enzymes can enable your body to return to its higher functioning condition of youth. In addition to these healing duties, enzymes also pull out the garbage from your cells for removal. On the one hand, this is a very exciting function because it means that years of bad eating and hard living can be reversed. On the other hand, it means that this garbage, when pulled out of your cells, is suddenly somewhere else in your body—namely, in your bloodstream and eliminative organs. If you transition carefully and ensure that the garbage is fully eliminated through increased bowel activity, sweat, deep breathing, massage, and adequate, gentle sunlight, you will gracefully and easily turn over a new body.

—*Natalia Rose,* The Raw Food Detox Diet

A steady intake of fresh fruit and vegetable juice will aid the cleansing process immensely. Green vegetable juice in particular is considered the lifeblood of a successful raw-food diet. The abundance of chlorophyll, organic minerals, and enzymes in green juice makes it rich in alkalinity, so it neutralizes the body's acidity. In addition to sending freshly oxygenated living cells into the bloodstream to recharge our blood, the chlorophyll works as an excellent blood builder, with magnesium as its central molecule.

As you know, a juicer separates the juice from the fiber of the fruits or vegetables so that we can ingest much more of the pure organic liquid (which contains all the vitamins, minerals, and enzymes) without the bulk of the fiber getting in the way and filling us up. This means that your body will not have to spend as much energy on digestion, and the enzymes and nutrients will go straight to the cellular level to do their cleansing work. If you do not have access to a juicer but do have a good blender, you can make raw smoothies and blended soups instead of the juices, but the cleansing effect will not be as pronounced. I strongly recommend that you buy or borrow a juicer for these three transformative weeks.

In addition to working with the food we take into our bodies, we also can use yoga, meditation, and breath work as vehicles for cleansing and gaining clarity. If you practice yoga, you already know about its power to transform us at the deepest level of our being:

Typically, we are unaware when we begin a yoga practice that we have vast reservoirs of energy and aliveness lying dormant within us. . . . Initially, we will notice positive changes just by moving our body in ways we never used to, and eventually, change occurs because we become more attuned to our breathing, energy rhythms, mind states, and innermost potential.

—*Sarah Powers*

Over these twenty-one days and ideally beyond, try to practice some yoga daily—and watch what happens. I also encourage you to commit to at least five minutes of meditation each and every day.

For your daily meditations, simply set a timer for five minutes or longer, find a comfortable seat on the floor (cross-legged or with your legs extended out in front of you), perhaps with your back resting against a wall for support. Close your eyes, tune into your breath, and observe your thoughts. You can do this several times during the day, but unless you already have a regular meditation practice, I suggest that you limit your meditation sessions to just five minutes. More specific instructions on meditation appear in Day One.

DAY ONE

Every twenty-four hour day is a tremendous gift to us. So we
all should learn to live in a way that makes joy and happiness
possible.

—Thich Nhat Hanh

As you embark on Day One of this twenty-one-day journey, I suggest that you take some time today to set your own personal intention for these next three weeks.

Consider how you would like to structure your transition. Would you like to adhere to the following timeline, or do you prefer to alter the timing to suit your needs:

Week 1: Eliminate all refined sugar and white flour.

Week 2: Also eliminate animal products.

Week 3: Also eliminate all cooked food and processed foods and eat 100 percent raw fruits and vegetables for the entire last week of the cleanse.

You also may want to review these guidelines and consider which of the following areas you want to focus on most:

❖ Drink lots of spring or distilled water.

❖ Start each day with a cup of hot water with lemon juice.

❖ Drink green lemonade and other fresh vegetable and fruit juices or smoothies.

❖ Eat as many raw fruits and vegetables as possible.

❖ Limit eating to the daylight hours.

❖ Eat only fresh fruits until noon.

❖ Always eat fruit by itself, separate from other foods.

❖ Rest and get plenty of sleep.

❖ Breathe using simple breathing techniques.

❖ Sweat with yoga, dance, or other exercise, a sauna, or a hot bath.

❖ Go outdoors for a walk, run, or bike ride.

❖ Practice yoga.

❖ Meditate for at least five minutes a day.

❖ Unplug from the television, computer, cell phone, and iPod.

❖ Be inspired by good books and music.

Please take the time to write your intention down in your own handwriting now and keep it in a place where you will see it often over the coming weeks. Your intention does not have to be long or elaborate—just a few phrase will do.

Perhaps you can use this example and fill in the blank with one or more of the phrases below:

As I embark on this cleanse, over the next three weeks I seek to _____.

—meditate every day

—spend some time outdoors each day

—do some yoga each and every day

—practice some simple breathing techniques to relax and live more fully in the present moment

—eat many more raw fruits and vegetables than I do now

—drink at least one fresh fruit or vegetable juice or smoothie every day

—eliminate sugar and refined flour from my diet

—eliminate animal products (i.e., meat, poultry, fish, dairy, and eggs) from my diet

—eat little or no cooked food for at least one full week

—be more present to my experience of each moment as it unfolds

—avoid watching television and movies unless they are truly enriching

—limit the time I spend on my cell phone and computer

—read something inspiring for at least a few minutes each day

—stop eating after sunset

—spend time observing beauty in nature, art, dance, theater, or film

—listen to classical music for a little while every day

—truly show up for the people in my life

—let myself be still and quiet

Exercise for Day One

THE THREE ARRIVALS—A BASIC MEDITATION TECHNIQUE

Find a quiet place where you can sit uninterrupted for at least five minutes. Take a comfortable seat, preferably on the floor. It can be helpful to sit on a cushion or a folded towel or blanket in order to lift your hips and relieve pressure on the lower back and pelvic region. You may choose to lean your back against a wall for additional support. Cross your legs loosely in front of you, or extend your legs straight out in front. Set a timer for just five minutes, and begin with a simple, traditional meditation technique called "The Three Arrivals":

First, *arrive with your body.* Bring your awareness into your body, and notice your physical sensations. Observe where you feel tightness or discomfort, and allow yourself to experience those feelings.

Second, *arrive with your breath.* Focus on your breath. Feel as though the breath is breathing you. Allow your breath to be easy and natural. Simply observe the breath.

Third, *arrive with the mind.* Notice the quality of your mental state. Is your mind racing? Are you distracted, or do you feel calm and centered? Watch what happens with your thoughts. Create some distance from them, as though they are moving across a movie screen. Simply witness your thoughts without thinking about the past or planning for the future. Settle into the present moment, and simply be aware.

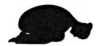

Yoga Pose for Day One

CHILD'S POSE (*BALASANA*)

Benefits: Gently stretches the hips, thighs, and ankles; calms the brain and helps to relieve stress and fatigue; relieves back and neck pain when done with head and torso supported.

Do not do this pose if you are pregnant or are recovering from a serious knee injury.

Kneel on the floor with your big toes and ankles touching. Sit back on your heels, You may separate your knees to hip width if you like. Place your chest and ribcage down onto your thighs. Rest your forehead on the mat, if possible.

Lay your hands on the floor alongside your torso, palms up, and release the fronts of your shoulders toward the floor. Feel how the weight of the front shoulders pulls the shoulder blades wide across your back. You also may want to try reaching your arms out in front of you on the floor.

Child's Pose is a resting pose, so you may stay for several minutes. Take deep, full breaths as your relax into this calming pose.

Beginning today and for the first week of the cleanse, I encourage you to eliminate all foods that contain refined sugar and processed flour, which means no bread, pasta, crackers, cookies, cake, or pastries. It also would be good to avoid caffeinated beverages such as coffee and black or green tea and alcoholic beverages. Alcohol, tea, and coffee tax the adrenal glands, create acidity in the body, and put a strain on the immune system.

This cleanse is designed to help you rid yourself of built-up toxins so that you can enjoy all the health and vitality that nature has to offer without being affected by the unnatural stimulation of sugary, caffeinated, or processed foods. Use this time to become more keenly attuned to your body's natural state without altering that state through the use of refined sugar, alcohol, or caffeine.

Daily Cleanse Regimen

Start today and every day with a cup of hot water with the fresh juice of one lemon stirred in. Drink several glasses of spring or distilled water throughout the morning. Do not rush to eat, and if possible, let the first thing you have each day be a glass of green lemonade made in a juicer. If you do not have a juicer, then you can use a blender and add some water to dilute the mixture.

. . . .

Green Lemonade

(Makes one 12-ounce serving)

1 head romaine lettuce or celery

5-6 stalks kale (preferably lacinato kale, which is also called "elephant kale" owing to its wrinkled, elephant skin appearance)

1 whole lemon

1-3 apples (I recommend Granny Smith or Fuji)—optional, as needed for sweetness

1-2 inches fresh ginger—optional

If possible, please use organic produce for this and all recipes in this book.

. . . .

Throughout the morning and up until noon, feel free to eat *as much fresh fruit as you like*, but skip other foods. Lunch and dinner can be whatever you like, but avoid sugar and flour, so no bread, pasta, crackers, or cookies. Try to start your lunch and dinner meals with a big salad. Remember to eat fruit by itself. After eating other types of food, allow at least three hours to pass before eating fruit. After you eat fruit, wait at least thirty minutes to eat other types of food.

Follow the sun: Do your best to refrain from eating after the sun sets. This will take some getting used to, especially because we tend to be in the habit of eating far into the evening. Having other things to do will help—you might try taking a walk or a bath after sundown or do some reading and climb into bed earlier than usual.

RECIPES FOR DAY ONE

* *

Fortifying Juice

6 oz carrot juice

1 oz beet juice

1 oz parsley or watercress juice

Juice all ingredients in a juicer and drink immediately.

* *

Detoxifying Green Smoothie

(Makes 1 quart)

½ bunch cilantro

1 cup stinging nettles

½ bunch fresh parsley

2 stalks celery

2 tablespoons lemon juice

1 mango

Blend all ingredients together in a blender until smooth.

* *

Creamy Raw Mushroom Soup

2 cups raw cashew milk (See recipe below.)

½ onion

1 clove garlic

1 cup mushrooms (cremini, portabello, or plain button mushrooms)

2 tablespoons Nama Shoyu soy sauce or Bragg's liquid aminos

1 tablespoon lime juice

Sea salt to taste

Extra mushrooms for garnish, diced

Process all ingredients in a blender or food processor until creamy. Top with extra diced mushrooms.

For the Raw Cashew Milk:

½ cup raw cashews, soaked for at least one hour, drained, and rinsed

2 cups water

1 tablespoon raw honey or raw agave syrup

Sea salt to taste

Blend soaked cashews and water in a blender for at least one minute. Add raw honey or raw agave nectar to taste. You may vary the amount of water to achieve the desired consistency. You also may choose to strain your raw cashew milk to remove the graininess.

* *

Lettuce and Persimmon Salad with Walnut Butter Dressing

1 head romaine lettuce, chopped

2 large Fuyu persimmons, chopped

½ large fennel bulb, sliced thinly

2 large handfuls of alfalfa sprouts

1 tablespoon hemp seeds—optional

Place all ingredients in a large bowl, and toss with walnut dressing.

For the Walnut Butter Dressing:

1 tablespoon walnut butter or any other raw nut butter of your choice

Juice from 1 large orange

Blend in a blender until smooth, or place in a jar and shake vigorously until combined.

* *

Zucchini Pasta

1 small to medium zucchini per person (You also may substitute rutabaga or turnip.)

Run the zucchini or other vegetable through a Saladacco shredder or food processor for long "spaghetti," or simply cut by hand into thin shreds.

Rinse and drain in a colander for a few minutes. Top with Italian Tomato Sauce or Pesto Sauce (see recipes below).

For the Italian Tomato Sauce:

3 large fresh vine-ripened organic tomatoes, ⅓ chopped into chunks, ⅔ pureed in blender or food processor

1 garlic clove, peeled and crushed

¼ cup fresh basil and oregano, mixed

1 tablespoon dried Italian herb mixture (including basil, oregano, thyme, and parsley)

Fresh ground black pepper to taste

¼ onion, minced

¼ cup extra-virgin olive oil

2 tablespoons raw apple cider vinegar

1 tablespoon raw honey or raw agave nectar

Dash of cinnamon

Blend all ingredients in blender until smooth. Serve over Zucchini Pasta.

For the Pesto Sauce:

½ bunch of fresh basil

½ cup pine nuts or walnuts, or a combination of both

1 clove fresh garlic, peeled and crushed

½ cup extra-virgin olive oil

Fresh black pepper to taste

Chop the basil together with the nuts for a few seconds in a food processor. Add all the remaining ingredients, and pulse into a thick, chunky paste. Serve tossed with Zucchini Pasta.

DAY TWO

When the mind is quiet, we come to know ourselves as the pure witness. We withdraw from the experience and its experiencer and stand apart in pure awareness, which is between and beyond the two.

—*Sri Nisargadatta Maharaj*

The practice of becoming the witness to our life experience is a potent exercise in gaining insight and perspective. On a regular basis, we need to step away from the busyness and distractions of our lives and draw more deeply into ourselves. As we allow our minds to grow quiet, we become more attentive observers, watching our thoughts and sensations and listening carefully to the stirrings of our heart. From this place of inner reflection, we are better able to recognize the tremendous gift of the body we inhabit.

Exercise for Day Two

REFLECT ON THE GIFT OF YOUR BODY

Take a few minutes to relax your body and your mind. Turn your attention to your breath. After a few moments, move your attention into your body. Feel its warmth, the sensations, your breathing, the air on your skin. Practice this meditation of body awareness for a few minutes.

Then take a moment to contemplate the gift of your body. Reflect on how your body has carried you through life, supported the experience of joy, and endured the experience of sorrow. Cultivate a feeling of gratitude toward your body. Consider the ways in which you take your body for granted. Ask yourself: *How can I be more kind to my body, which has been a faithful friend to me?*

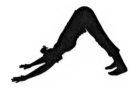

Yoga Pose for Day Two

DOWNWARD-FACING DOG POSE (*ADHO MUKHA SVANASANA*)

Benefits: Stretches all the muscles in the back, belly, shoulders, calves, and thighs; strengthens arms; stimulates abdominal organs; and relieves neck tension and relaxes general tension.

Find a quiet place. Begin in a tabletop position on all fours with your palms directly under your shoulders and your hips over your knees. Curl your toes under, and lift the knees up several inches off the floor. Press your ribcage back toward your thighs, and slowly begin to straighten your knees as you lift your tailbone upward to form an inverted V with your body. Once your knees are straight, gently lower your heels down to the floor, coming into Downward-Facing Dog Pose.

Draw your navel up toward your spine. Keep your arms and legs straight, with your feet parallel, so that your heels do not turn inward or outward. Remain here for several minutes, listening to your breath and finding extension through your spine and along the backs of your legs. When you are ready, simply bend your knees and bring them down to the mat, pause in a tabletop position before coming to sit on the mat for several minutes with your eyes closed, experiencing the effects of this classic yoga pose. Hold for five to ten breaths, and gently come down to rest in the Child's Pose.

During the first week of the cleanse, you will be eliminating foods that contain refined sugar and flour, as well as alcohol and caffeine. Although white flour is the biggest culprit, all types of processed flour will behave like glue in your digestive tract and greatly impede the cleansing action of the raw fruits, vegetables, and juices you are adding to your diet. To get maximum benefit from the cleanse, it is best to eliminate all types of flour, including whole wheat, rice, spelt, quinoa, rye, barley, and oat flour. This means that you will be avoiding all pastas, breads, crackers, cookies, and cakes. Moving away from processed foods and toward a more whole foods–based diet will bring you vibrant health. Eating food in its pure, unaltered form helps us to recognize and appreciate its natural beauty and to feel a deeper connection to nature.

With the elimination of sugar and flour, you may have cravings for starchy foods. While you want to stay away from all types of flour, cooked whole grains such as millet, brown rice, and quinoa are acceptable options, especially during this first week of the cleanse. Whole grains could remain a part of your diet, even into the second week, when we will be eliminating animal products. During the last week of the cleanse, though, I encourage you to eat a 100 percent raw-food diet of fruits, vegetables, and fresh juices, as well as moderate amounts of nuts and seeds. You will achieve optimal cleansing results if you cut out all cooked foods, including cooked grains during that final week. If you want to move ahead more quickly, you may start to reduce your intake of animal products and cooked foods as soon as you like.

Otherwise, for now, it is fine to include cooked whole grains in your diet, perhaps trying to limit them more and more as the cleanse progresses. You also might consider some raw-food options that will curb your starch cravings—such as bananas and rich, sweet fruits such as mangos, as well as soaked nuts and seeds for their density. Above all, please be patient with yourself. If you are accustomed to a cooked-food diet containing lots of starchy foods, then it is going to take you some time to adjust to all this lighter fare.

DETOXIFICATION SYMPTOMS

If caffeine, alcohol, and sugar are a regular feature of your diet, then in these first few days of the cleanse you will already be experiencing the discomfort of withdrawal from these stimulating substances. The initial days of detoxification can be extremely challenging, and I want to remind you to be patient. The detox symptoms are likely to subside within a few days, and you will feel so much better. But I also want to remind you to be kind to yourself. If you are feeling overwhelmed by the withdrawal symptoms, you can choose to make a more gradual transition away from caffeine.

Much of the power of a raw-food cleanse lies in it's effect on the body's pH. The pH of our blood is naturally slightly alkaline, but if we eat a highly acidic diet, our body has to work extra hard to keep its blood pH constant. Coffee and black tea are extremely acidic, even in decaffeinated form, so they greatly hinder the cleansing process. Caffeine also causes dehydration and taxes the kidneys, causing loss of calcium and a host of other problems, including anxiety, sleep disruptions, restlessness, irritability, brain fog, indecision, bloating, and feeling cold.

The negative effects of caffeine may give you ample motivation to limit or avoid coffee and black tea altogether. However, since caffeine is so addictive, eliminating it all at once can have a dramatic detox effect, including severe headaches, irritability, flu symptoms, and so on that can last from a few days to an entire week. Cutting back more gradually will alleviate the withdrawal symptoms. If you drink coffee, you can begin by replacing the caffeinated coffee with one-half decaf and also reduce your overall coffee intake a little bit each day over the course of a week or so. If you are drinking caffeinated tea, you can dip the tea bag in warm water first to release most of the caffeine before steeping it to drink and gradually replace your caffeinated tea with an herbal alternative.

Herbal teas are an excellent substitute for coffee or caffeinated tea. Any of the packaged herbal teas are fine, but it also can be wonderful to make your own tea from loose herbs that are often available in bulk at health food stores. Several homemade herbal tea recipes are included here in today's recipes.

Sugar can perform like a drug in your system, creating a temporary "high" of energy and elevating your mood. If you typically consume a lot of sugar, a sudden attempt to eliminate it may leave you feeling irritable, with low energy, cravings for sugar-loaded foods, and even headaches and flu-like symptoms. With both caffeine and sugar withdrawal, it is helpful to drink as much water as possible and to use plenty of raw fruits, vegetables, and fresh homemade juices to help flush the body of the toxins that are being released. You also can feel free to satisfy your sweet tooth with extrasweet fruits such as mangos, bananas, and figs. Fresh is much better than dried, but it is fine to indulge in a little bit of unsweetened dried fruit if that helps stave off the cravings during the transition period. Please note that dried fruit is much easier to digest and much more cleansing if it is soaked in water for several hours. Be patient, and try to ride out any discomfort at this point. Your detoxification symptoms will soon pass.

RECIPES FOR DAY TWO

Lemon-Lime Ginger Ale

Handful of grapes

1 apple, cored and sliced

½ inch fresh ginger (less if you find the taste too strong)

½ lime

¼ lemon

Sparkling mineral water

Remove the grapes from the stem. Juice the apple and ginger together, and then juice the rest of the fruit. Pour the juice into a large glass, fill to the top with sparkling water, and serve with ice.

Super Green Smoothie

(Makes 1 quart)

2 leaves kale, stems removed

2 leaves chard, stems removed

¼ cup fresh parsley

1 small leaf aloe vera

¼ cup dandelion greens

1 pear

1 banana

1½ cups water

Blend all ingredients together in a blender until smooth.

· ·

Miso Soup

5 brazil nuts

2 strips kelp, soaked in warm water until soft

2 tablespoons coconut oil—optional

1 teaspoon Ume plum paste—optional

2 teaspoons curry powder

1 teaspoon fresh ginger, grated

1 clove garlic, minced

3 tablespoons unpasteurized miso

4 cups water

1 small chili, minced, or a dash of cayenne pepper

½ cup carrots, roughly chopped

Blend all ingredients in a blender until smooth and creamy.

· ·

Creamy Asian Salad

(Makes 2 to 4 servings)

For the Salad:

1 cup mung bean sprouts

1 cup shredded green or purple cabbage

½ red bell pepper, thinly sliced

½ cup sugar snap peas

¼ cup mushrooms (shitake or button), sliced

2 tablespoons fresh cilantro, chopped

1 tablespoon fresh basil, chopped

½ clove garlic, chopped

Mix all ingredients together, and set aside.

For the Dressing:

½ inch ginger, chopped

½ cup cold-pressed olive oil

1 teaspoon sesame oil

1 clove garlic

2 tablespoons lemon juice

3 whole dates, pitted

1 tablespoon Nama Shoyu soy sauce

2 tablespoons water

Blend all ingredients in a blender until smooth. One hour before serving, pour half the dressing over the salad. Mix thoroughly.

* *

Raw Sushi

(Makes 8 rolls)

2 sheets nori seaweed

2 romaine leaves

½ cup alfalfa sprouts

½ cucumber, julienned

½ carrot, shredded or julienned

½ avocado, sliced—optional

Place the nori sheet in front of you. Lay one leaf of romaine lettuce horizontally on the top of the nori sheet on the side closest to you. Lay the sprouts, cucumber pieces, and carrot pieces horizontally following the line of the romaine leaf. Carefully roll it tightly. Moisten the end of the nori farthest from you with water, and seal it like an envelope. Slice the roll with a sharp knife down the middle, or cut it into smaller one- to two-inch pieces.

For the Japanese "Rice":

(Makes about 1 cup)

½ cup chopped parsnips

¼ cup raw pine nuts

1 tablespoon raw honey

⅓ tablespoon rice vinegar

1 tablespoon raw teriyaki sauce (see below)

Pulse the parsnips, pine nuts, honey, and vinegar in a food processor until the mixture resembles brown rice. Add the sauce, and mix well. Serve alongside Raw Sushi (above).

For the Teriyaki Sauce:

¼ cup Nama Shoyu soy sauce

¼ cup raw agave nectar

¼ teaspoon ginger, whole

½ teaspoon minced garlic

1 drizzle sesame oil

Blend all the ingredients in a blender, and use as a dipping sauce.

* *

DAY THREE

The discipline of yoga is a purification practice, but not in the sense that we [are] inclined to believe. The goal is purification not for the sake of perfection but for the sake of freedom. . . . Rather than struggling against a pose, you can relax into it and receive the gift of opening it has to offer.

—Kate Tremblay

It is excellent to use your yoga practice to facilitate the cleanse on both the physical and mental fronts. If you can attend yoga classes frequently over these twenty-one days, that is wonderful. But whether you go to yoga class or not, it is immensely helpful to do some yoga on your own at home, preferably a little bit each day. While yoga classes provide encouragement and motivation, you are always your own best teacher, and a personal home yoga practice will give you invaluable insight into yourself. Try to do a few yoga poses on your own every day, even if it is just for ten to twenty minutes. As with meditation, it is helpful to build your personal yoga practice into your early-morning routine if possible. You will be amazed at how a few yoga poses will help to set the tone for your day.

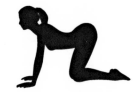

Yoga Pose for Day Three
CAT/COW POSE
Benefits: Stretches the front torso and neck, and provides a gentle massage to the spine and abdominal organs.

If you have a neck injury, keep your head in line with your torso. Begin in a tabletop position, with your knees under your hips and your shoulders directly above your wrists. Look straight down at the floor so that the neck is long. As you exhale, round your spine toward the ceiling, making sure to keep your shoulders and knees in position. Release your head toward the floor, and experience a stretch across the shoulder blades. This is the Cat Pose.

As you inhale, lift your tailbone and chest toward the ceiling, allowing your belly to sink toward the floor. Lift and open your chest. Let your head fall back slightly, coming into the Cow Pose. Alternate between the Cat and Cow Pose five to ten times.

THE PHILOSOPHY OF YOGA

Initially, the discipline of hatha yoga—the physical aspect of yoga—was developed as a vehicle for meditation. The repertoire of hatha yoga prepared the body, and particularly the nervous system, for stillness, creating the necessary physical strength and stamina that allowed the mind to remain calm.

While the physical practice of yoga has gained popularity in recent years, the philosophical underpinnings of yoga remain largely underexposed. Classical yoga is a philosophical system that has its roots in ancient India. Yoga comes from a Sanskrit word that has several translations and can be interpreted in many ways. It derives from the root *yug* and originally meant "to hitch up," as in attaching horses to a vehicle. Another definition is "to put to active and purposeful use." Still other translations are "to yoke, join, or concentrate."

In essence, yoga has come to describe a means of uniting or a method of discipline. The practice of yoga grew out of an oral tradition in which the teaching was transmitted directly from teacher to student. The Indian sage Patanjali has been credited with the collation of this oral tradition into his classical work, *Yoga Sutra*, a 2,000-year-old treatise on yogic philosophy that generally is accepted as the ultimate source book of classical yoga. In this revered text, Patanjali, who is thought to have been a physician, Sanskrit scholar, and yogi, presents astanga yoga, or an "eight-limbed path" of practice.

The path begins with ten ethical precepts called *yamas* (restraints) and *niyamas* (observances). The *five yamas* that comprise the *first limb* of yoga are

ahimsa (nonharming)
satya (truthfulness)
asteya (nonstealing)
brahmacharya (clarity about sexual activity)
aparigraha (nongreed)

The *five niyamas* that make up the *second limb* are

shauca (purity)
santosha (contentment)
tapas (discipline)
svadhyaya (self-study)
ishivara pranidhana (surrender to God)

The *third and fourth limbs* are *asana* (posture) and *pranayama* (breath control). The *fifth limb* is *pratyahara* (the conscious withdrawal from the agitation of the senses). The *sixth limb* is *dharana* (concentration), the *seventh limb* is *dhyana* (meditation), and the *eighth limb* is *samadhi* (oneness). Taken together, these eight limbs help you to develop self-awareness.

As you practice the physical aspect of yoga, the *asanas*, you might consider the philosophical context from which they developed and reflect on how the philosophy of yoga relates to your life.

RECIPES FOR DAY THREE

* *

Potassium Drink

4 medium carrots, greens removed
1 stalk celery
1 apple
Handful of fresh parsley
Handful of fresh spinach
½ lemon, peeled—optional
Juice all ingredients in a juicer, and drink immediately.

* *

Watermelon-Lime Smoothie

(Makes 1 quart)

½ small watermelon
2 limes, juiced
Blend all ingredients together in a blender until smooth.

* *

Cream of Cauliflower Soup

(Makes 1 to 2 servings)

1 cup cauliflower
1 cup water
¼ cup raw cashews or pine nuts
1 tablespoon lemon juice
Sea salt to taste
Blend all ingredients in a blender until thick and smooth.

* *

Shaved Asparagus Salad with Mustard Seed

(Makes 2 servings)

½ bunch asparagus
5 radishes, sliced thin
⅓ cup fresh orange juice
2 tablespoons apple cider vinegar
½ teaspoon mustard seed

¼ cup extra-virgin olive oil

Sea salt and freshly ground black pepper to taste

1 tablespoon orange zest

Wash asparagus and trim ends. Cut off asparagus tips and set to the side. Shave the asparagus bracts with a vegetable peeler.

For the Mustard Seed Vinaigrette:

Blend vinegar, olive oil, mustard seeds, and orange juice in a blender until smooth.

For the Assembly:

Toss together the shaved asparagus, sliced radishes, coarse pepper, sea salt, and vinaigrette. Garnish with asparagus tips and orange zest.

* *

Endive Bruschetta

(Makes about 5 servings)

1 Roma tomato, diced

½ clove garlic, minced

¼ cup packed fresh basil

Sea salt and freshly ground black pepper to taste

½ head endive, separated into leaves

Combine the tomato, garlic, basil, salt, and pepper. Place a heaping tablespoon of the mixture on each endive leaf.

* *

DAY FOUR

May wisdom fully awaken in your heart and in your mind.
—*Anonymous*

As we cultivate awareness, we are drawn away from our thoughts about the past or the future and toward a more authentic experience of the present moment. The more we can develop an ability to simply be present, the closer we come to wisdom. This is so because our wisdom nature is self-revealing. The mere act of being awake and aware in the moment allows our innate wisdom to emerge on its own. This inner wisdom is not something that is acquired from somewhere outside ourselves, nor is it a quality that must be achieved over a long period of time. Rather, it is an inherent element of our being that has always been there, a kind of primordial "knowing."

As you move toward a more genuine, wakeful way of living, your wisdom nature will become more apparent and accessible.

Exercise for Day Four

RECOGNIZING YOUR WISDOM NATURE

In a quiet place, ask yourself: *When have I felt truly content and at peace within?* Call to mind a time in your life when you have felt calm and centered, perhaps recently or even at some point in your childhood. Bring yourself back to that memory, and relive the feeling of being grounded and at ease.

The "deeper self" that revealed itself to you then in that moment of peace and stability never really goes away. Perhaps at times, though, the distractions and complexities of life lead you away from that sense of serenity and inner fulfillment. If you feel that you have lost touch with your innermost essence, remind yourself that although often shrouded in the veil of confusion and ignorance, your innermost essence is indeed always present.

Each one of us has a wisdom nature, and each of us senses it at a deep level. Regardless of your life circumstances and the course that your relationships have taken, you possess a reservoir of inner wisdom.

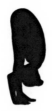

Yoga Pose for Day Four

STANDING-FORWARD FOLD (*UTTANASANA*)

Benefits: Stretches the hamstrings, calves, lower back, and neck. Quiets the mind and calms the nervous system after a stressful time or at the end of a busy day.

Do not practice this pose if you have glaucoma or retinal problems, sciatica, disk disease, a head cold, or a sinus headache. Stand with your feet one foot apart, your feet parallel, and your knees straight. Place your hands on your hips. As you exhale, hinge at your hips and bend forward from the hip joints, keeping your spine long and extended. You may bend your knees slightly if you feel a strain in your lower back as you come forward.

Once you are far enough forward, lightly place your fingertips on the floor in line with your toes. Gently drop your head forward, perhaps nodding yes and no several times to release tension in the neck and shoulders. Allow gravity to lengthen your spine as the weight of your head draws you forward. Feel free to keep the knees soft and slightly bent if you feel too much strain in your lower back.

Take five to ten deep, relaxed breaths. As you inhale, bend your knees slightly, and let your head hang as your roll up through your spine to come to standing.

As you move to a more whole foods–based diet and use raw foods to cleanse your system, it is helpful to consider the transit time of foods through your body. The most cleansing foods for the body are the easiest foods to digest, and they leave your body quickly. These foods are referred to as *quick-exit foods*, foods that pass through the body rapidly, leaving the least amount of reside behind that can turned into waste matter and create toxicity in your system. Hydrating fresh fruits and vegetables top the list of quick-exit foods.

QUICK-EXIT HIERARCHY OF FOOD (1 = BEST, 11 = WORST)

1. Raw fruits and vegetables (preferably organic), such as apples, grapes, melons, bananas, avocados, romaine lettuce, cucumbers, carrots, kale, and tomatoes, and raw honey and stevia

2. Lightly steamed low-starch vegetables (all vegetables other than white potatoes, acorn and butternut squash, and pumpkin), pure maple syrup, and agave nectar
3. Raw nuts and seeds, such as almonds, pine nuts, walnuts, macadamia nuts, sunflower seeds, and sesame seeds
4. Raw cold-pressed plant oils, especially olive oil and flax seed oil
5. Cooked starchy vegetables such as sweet potatoes, butternut squash, acorn squash, and pumpkin
6. Whole grains such as brown rice, millet, whole wheat, and buckwheat
7. Raw unpasteurized dairy products from goats and sheep
8. Pasteurized dairy and animal flesh
9. All flour products, such as bread, white rice, pasta, crackers, flour tortillas, cookies, and cakes, and sugar (both white and brown sugar)
10. Cooked animal fats/hydrogenated oils, mainstream meats, poultry, and soy products
11. Chemicals, artificial sweeteners (aspartame, saccharine), and unnatural additives

Throughout the cleanse, it is best to eat foods that fall within levels 1 to 6 of the quick-exit hierarchy. It is ideal if you can have the level 1 foods dominate your diet. This means eating as many fresh fruits and vegetables as you can and drinking homemade juices as often as possible. While there is no need to rush ahead to a predominantly raw-food diet, it is extremely helpful to eat as much raw produce as possible to crowd out the less healthy stuff—such as the cooked foods and animal products. You can choose to see this as chance to indulge in lots of raw, living foods rather than feeling as though you are restricting or depriving yourself.

If you can begin each day with plenty of water and a big serving of green lemonade (over time, increasing the amount to 40 ounces each day) and then eat some fresh fruit until noon, you will be off to an excellent start. As the day goes on, you might add heavier foods, always starting off with a big salad and then perhaps some cooked whole foods such as steamed or sautéed vegetables and whole grains or a soup.

This approach is referred to as *eating light to heavy*. We start with the lightest foods, the ones that pass through our system the fastest (see the quick-exit hierarchy above) and gradually move to denser, slower-moving foods as the day progresses. If you eat something that takes several hours to pass through your digestive tract and exit the body and then eat a quick-moving food on top of that, the fast-exit food is going to get held up by the slower-exit food, and the result will be fermentation and an overall slowing down of digestion and elimination, which will impede the cleanse and make you feel pretty awful.

Please remember to listen to your body and, most of all, to your inner wisdom at every stage of the cleanse.

RECIPES FOR DAY FOUR

- -

Pear-Kale-Mint Juice

4 ripe pears

5 kale leaves

½ bunch mint

2 cups water

Juice all ingredients in a juicer, and drink immediately.

- -

Kale-Tomato-Basil Green Smoothie

(Makes 1 quart)

5 kale leaves

½ bunch fresh dill

½ lime, juiced

3 cloves garlic—optional

¼ cup sun-dried tomatoes

2 cups water

Blend all ingredients in a blender until smooth.

- -

Honeydew-Cucumber Soup

(Makes 2 servings)

½ honeydew melon, peeled and chopped

½ cucumber, peeled, seeded, and sliced

Several sprigs of mint, stems removed

Blend the cucumber and mint in a blender, add the melon, and blend on low speed. Chill and serve.

- -

· ·

Green Salad with Cucumbers and Mangoes

2–3 hearts or ½ large head of romaine lettuce, torn into bite-sized pieces

2–3 baby cucumbers or ½ large cucumber, sliced

2–3 mangoes, cubed

3–4 medium tomatoes, diced

½ cup cilantro, chopped

Combine all ingredients, toss, and serve.

· ·

Indian Curry Vegetables

(Makes 2 to 3 servings)

4 apricots, sliced (or 2–3 dates, pits removed), soaked for twenty to thirty minutes

¼ cup warm water

3 cups assorted chopped vegetables, such as cauliflower, broccoli, zucchini, carrots, green beans, red bell peppers, collard greens, or spinach

2 tablespoons minced spring onion, red onion, or other onion

1 tablespoon minced ginger

1 clove garlic

¼ teaspoon curry powder

¼ teaspoon coriander

¼ teaspoon sea salt

½ tablespoon Nama Shoyu soy sauce

2 tablespoons minced cilantro

Soak apricots or dates in ¼ cup warm water for twenty minutes. Toss all the vegetables together. Place the remaining ingredients, except the cilantro, in a blender or food processor along with the apricots (or dates) and the soaking water. Process on high speed for thirty seconds or as long as it takes to blend the apricots (or dates) into a thick paste. Toss the vegetables together with the spiced sauce. Allow the vegetables to marinate for several hours before serving.

· ·

DAY
FIVE

Do not be afraid to leave your old habits behind long enough
to try on new ones. If you admire someone, let the sage in that
person inspire the sage in you.

—Lama Miller

Our admiration of others gives us a tangible starting place for our own growth and development. It can be helpful to identify several people whom you admire and then to reflect on the character traits that inspire you. You even may choose to write those qualities down: words such as *integrity, kindness, patience, fortitude, courage,* and *wisdom*. Once you define the traits that you would like to develop in yourself, take small steps toward emulating them in your daily life.

Exercise for Day Five

SEEING YOUR INNATE QUALITIES

Sit in a quiet place. Think of a person you admire. What is one quality you value in that person? Patience? Generosity? Determination? Now think of a time when you manifested that quality yourself, even just a little. Acknowledge the seed potential of that quality within your own nature. Appreciate its presence, and know that if you nurture it, it will grow and flourish for you.

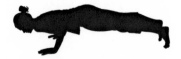

Yoga Pose for Day Five

UPPER AND LOWER PLANK POSE (*CHATURANGA*)

Benefits: Strengthens the arms and the muscles of the upper torso (the triceps and pectorals), engages the abdominal muscles, and develops core strength.

Do not do this pose if you are suffering from a wrist injury; take special care if you are recovering from a shoulder injury.

Upper plank: Come to your hands and knees. As you exhale, step your feet back to an upper push-up position, with your feet about six to eight inches apart, toes curled under. Create a long, straight line from your shoulders to your feet; ensure that your hips are in line with your shoulders and that your head does not drop below shoulder level. Hold for three to five full, steady breaths. You may bend your knees and bring them to the mat at any time if holding this pose feels like a strain.

Lower plank: From the upper plank position (see above), bring your shoulders and chest forward over your wrists, draw your elbows in close to your ribcage as you bend your arms, and slowly lower yourself to the floor, allowing the chin, chest, belly, and hips to land simultaneously. You can make this pose more challenging by taking a longer time to lower all the way down to the floor and even by letting yourself hover just a few inches above the floor before lowering completely down to rest on your mat.

THE MOST IMPORTANT FOODS TO BUY ORGANIC

While there has been some debate about whether organically grown food is more nutritious than conventionally grown food, we do not buy organic foods simply because they have more vitamins or minerals but also because of what they do not have—chemicals and pesticides. The Environmental Working Group (EWG), a nonprofit organization dedicated to consumer health and protection, regularly publishes the famous "Dirty Dozen," a listing of the foods most contaminated by pesticides. These are the foods that you should try to buy organic if possible. While the cost to our health of daily exposure to these chemicals has not been determined, it makes sense to try to limit our exposure if we can. Since organic food tends to be more expensive, it helps to know which foods are most likely to be contaminated so that you can prioritize.

Following is the EWG's updated list of the "Dirty Dozen," as well as its updated list for the "Clean Fifteen." The EWG posits that you can reduce your exposure to pesticides by up to 80 percent by buying the organic version of the "Dirty Dozen."

The Dirty Dozen

1. *Celery.* Since celery has no protective skin, you cannot wash off the chemicals. (Sixty-four chemicals have been identified in celery.)
2. *Peaches.* Sixty-two pesticides have been identified on these fruits.
3. *Strawberries.* Strawberries have long been on the list because they are one of the most sprayed crops on the planet. The EWG identified fifty-nine pesticides on strawberries.
4. *Apples.* While most of the forty-two different pesticides found on apples are concentrated on the skin, the skin is also the source of an awful lot of the beneficial nutrients in apples, so it is best not to peel them.
5. *Blueberries.* Unfortunately, this wonderful berry made the list for the first time. Blueberries are treated with up to fifty-two different pesticides.
6. *Nectarines.* Nectarines now rank with apples and peaches as the "dirtiest" of the tree fruits.
7. *Bell peppers.* Bell peppers are heavily sprayed with insecticides (as many as forty-nine on sweet bell peppers).
8. *Spinach.* Another new addition to the list for 2010, spinach can contain as many as forty-eight different chemicals, giving it the dubious honor of being the "dirtiest" green leafy vegetable around.
9. *Kale.* One of the healthiest vegetables on earth, kale also tested as one of the highest in pesticide residue.
10. *Cherries.* Government testing found forty-two different pesticides on cherries, and sadly, those grown in the United States seem to have three times more pesticide residue than imported cherries.
11. *Potatoes.* Back on the list after a year' s absence, the popular potato can have as many as thirty-seven different pesticides.
12. *Grapes.* Imported grapes seem to be the worst. No amount of washing will get rid of the residue.

The "Clean Fifteen" are the foods with the lowest pesticide residue. These are relatively safe to eat in their inorganic variety:

1. Onions
2. Avocados
3. Sweet corn
4. Pineapple
5. Mangos
6. Sweet peas
7. Asparagus
8. Kiwi
9. Cabbage
10. Eggplant

11. Cantaloupe
12. Watermelon
13. Grapefruit
14. Sweet potato
15. Honeydew melon

RECIPES FOR DAY FIVE

Sunshine Juice

4 granny smith apples or Gravenstein apples

2 inch fresh ginger, peeled

1 Meyer lemon, peeled

4 oz water to dilute

Juice all ingredients in a juicer, and drink immediately.

Pear Smoothie

(Makes 1 quart)

1 d'Anjou pear

3 leaves purple kale, stems removed

1 small leaf aloe vera

1 banana

Blend all ingredients together in a blender until smooth.

Green Spinach Soup

(Makes 2 servings)

1 avocado

1 red bell pepper

3 tablespoons fresh cilantro

1 cup spinach

1 lemon, seeded

1 cup of water

½ small jalapeno pepper

¼ teaspoon sea salt—optional

Blend all ingredients in a blender until creamy. Garnish with thinly sliced napa cabbage, red cabbage, or dulse leaves or flakes.

Classic Chopped Salad

(Makes 2 servings)

½ cup fresh green beans

2 ears fresh corn, kernels cut from cob

½ yellow bell pepper, chopped

1 large carrot, chopped

1 cup grape tomatoes, sliced in half

½ zucchini, chopped

1 tablespoon fresh chives, minced

2 tablespoons fresh lemon juice

½ teaspoon fresh garlic, diced

Blend all ingredients in a blender until smooth.

• •

Raw Ravioli

(Makes 16 raviolis)

1 large turnip, peeled

1 tablespoon extra-virgin olive oil

½ cup pine nuts, soaked for at least two hours

1 cup macadamia nuts, soaked for at least two hours

2 teaspoons fresh rosemary, minced

2 teaspoons fresh parsley, minced

2 teaspoons fresh thyme, minced

1 tablespoon nutritional yeast

½ teaspoon salt

½ teaspoon freshly ground black pepper

2 teaspoons apple cider vinegar

¼ cup water as needed

Using a vegetable peeler, a mandoline, or a sharp knife, cut turnips into sixteen very thin slices. Coat turnip slices in olive oil, and allow to marinate for at least one hour. Rinse pine nuts and macadamia nuts, and drain well for at least ten minutes. Place in a food processor fitted with an S-shaped blade, and process on high speed for ten seconds. Add rosemary, parsley, thyme, nutritional yeast, sea salt, black pepper, and apple cider vinegar. Blend on high speed for about twenty seconds while adding water through the top until you reach a smooth, cheesy consistency. Scoop 1 tablespoon of this mixture onto each turnip slice, and fold the slice in half. Cover with Sun-Dried Tomato-Sage Sauce (see recipe below).

For the Sun-Dried Tomato-Sage Sauce:

(Makes 1 cup)

2–3 tablespoons sun-dried tomatoes, chopped and soaked in ½ cup water

½ cup filtered water

1 cup Roma tomatoes, chopped

1 tablespoon beets, shredded

1 tablespoon extra-virgin olive oil

2 teaspoons fresh basil, minced

2 teaspoons fresh parsley, minced

½ teaspoon Nama Shoyu soy sauce

½ teaspoon nutritional yeast

¼ teaspoon fresh oregano, minced

¼ teaspoon fresh thyme, minced

¼ teaspoon sea salt

Pinch of freshly ground black pepper

1 teaspoon rubbed sage

Raw agave nectar to taste

Soak sun-dried tomatoes in ½ cup of water for at least thirty minutes. Drain and reserve liquid. Blend sun-dried tomatoes, Roma tomatoes, soak water, beets, olive oil, basil, parsley, Nama Shoyu soy sauce, nutritional yeast, oregano, thyme, salt, pepper, and sage in a blender to desired consistency.

● ●

DAY SIX

Yoga, like life itself, begins with the breath. Slow, steady, joyous breathing from the depths of our lungs oxygenates our blood, purifying our prana, chi, or life force. Breathe deeply, my friend, for breath is the key which awakens our powerful and true nature.

—*Duncan Wong*

Breathing is said to be the essence of mindfulness. As we seek to grow more awake and aware, we can use the breath as a bridge between our bodies and our minds. Often we are disconnected from our physical experience and lost in our thoughts about the past or the future. Memories and expectations cloud our perception and hinder our ability to be fully present to each moment as it unfolds. Establishing and then maintaining a connection with our breath helps us to touch life deeply in the here and now.

Throughout your day, you may choose to turn to your breath and allow it to bring you into a more authentic presence. In as few as ten to twenty seconds, your focus on your breath will radically transform your mental and physical state. You also may bring some breath work into your meditation sessions or your yoga practice,. Let your breath be the essential element and guiding force behind your practice. As your mind wanders, gently bring yourself back to the breath a thousand times. Over weeks and months, you will gradually learn to calm and center yourself using the breath.

Exercise for Day Six

FOLLOWING THE BREATH

Sit comfortably in a peaceful place. Notice your physical sensations without judging or criticizing.

Next, turn your awareness to your breath. Inhale naturally and normally. Continue in this way for three or four breaths.

Now follow your breath. Watch carefully as you draw the air in. Notice your sensations as you inhale. Track your outbreath, conscious of how the air exits your body. Continue to follow your breath for several minutes, maintaining a singular focus on the movement of the breath.

Begin to count your natural inhalations and exhalations. Most of us will take four to five counts to inhale and four to five counts to exhale. Next, simply inhale normally to a count of four or five, but elongate your exhalation to six to eight counts. Lengthening out your exhalations has a calming effect. It is helpful to use this technique when you are feeling anxious or stressed.

Conversely, you can stretch out your inhalations to six to eight counts, drawing the air in slowly, while exhaling for the normal four to five counts. Extending your inhalations is an uplifting practice and is beneficial at times when you are feeling insecure, fearful, or lacking in confidence.

This breathing exercise takes as little as ten to twenty seconds and may be done just about anywhere, anytime.

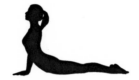

Yoga Pose for Day Six

COBRA POSE (*BHUJANGASANA*)

Benefits: Strengthens the muscles that line the spine, helps to improve posture, stretches the abdominal muscles and opens the chest, and increases flexibility in the upper and middle (thoracic and lumbar) spine, especially helpful after sitting for an extended period of time.

Do not do this pose after the first trimester of pregnancy. Be especially mindful when coming into this pose if you have diagnosed disk disease, spondylolysis, or spondylolisthesis.

Lie on your belly with your palms on the floor directly under your shoulders. Draw your elbows in close to your body. As you inhale, squeeze your shoulder blades together as you draw them down toward your waist. Press lightly down into your palms, and extend your chest forward. Avoid crunching in the neck and shoulders. Tuck your chin slightly into your chest so that your neck remains long. Allow your navel to remain on the floor, but lift it in and up toward your spine so that you are engaging your abdominal muscles slightly. Stay for three to five breaths, and gently lower your chest and chin down as you exhale. Repeat the pose several times.

If you have been able to reduce or eliminate your intake of refined sugar and processed flour this week, then already you have made great strides. Even if the shifts in your diet and daily routine have been subtle, I encourage you to look back on the past six days with gratitude for the positive changes you have adopted and also to look forward with eagerness and anticipation for what lies ahead. These next two weeks will be transformational.

Tomorrow begins the next phase of the cleanse, which involves eliminating animal products—meat, poultry, fish, dairy, and eggs—and consuming only plant-based foods. Ideally, you are already incorporating much more raw fruit, vegetables, and fresh juices and smoothies into your daily diet and letting those cleansing foods replace the less optimal choices such as bread, pasta, crackers, cookies, and cakes. As you prepare for this next phase, I want to discourage you from using imitation meat and cheese products. Those soy- or grain-based "meats" and "cheeses" are highly processed and take their ingredients so far away from their natural state.

ABOUT SOY

You might be surprised to learn that soy is the most mucus-forming food on the planet. It generates sticky, sludge-like mucus matter in your system that slows down the body's digestive flow and accumulates in your respiratory and digestive systems, creating asthmatic distress and digestive problems such as irritable bowel syndrome (IBS). You may be wondering about all the talk linking the predominance of soy in the Japanese diet to the good overall health of the Japanese people. It is helpful to note that the healthy Japanese diet actually includes much less soy than we think. The Japanese do not eat all the heavily processed soy foods that Americans consume, such as imitation chicken and meat. Rather, they eat edamame pods (soy in its natural, unprocessed state) and a small amount of tofu.

I advise you to limit your use of processed soy products such as tofu, soy milk, and so on. A little bit of tofu or soy milk will be fine, and small amounts of soy sauce or raw miso in recipes will not pose a problem. But too much heavily processed soy-based food will slow down your cleanse and lower the state of your overall health.

Rather than using overly processed dairy and meat substitutes, it is much better to focus on whole foods–based vegan meals that include fresh vegetables and some beans and whole grains. You also can use nuts and seeds in moderation, but please try to soak them for at least a few hours first to make them easier to digest. Nut and seed milks offer an excellent way to get the nutrition of nuts and seeds in a more easily assimilated form. Included below are several recipes for homemade nut and seed milks that you can make yourself in your blender or food processor.

In considering whether a food is truly healthful, a good rule of thumb is to ask yourself: Is this food in its natural state, and is its source recognizable? A tofu hotdog looks pretty different from a bright green soy bean pod, and a power bar does not look much like a fruit or a vegetable.

Again, instead of focusing on what you cannot have this week as you cleanse, such as meat or dairy products, focus on everything you *can* have—a large variety of fruits, vegetables, nuts, and seeds—all those rich colors and textures.

RECIPES FOR DAY SIX

* *

Fennel Juice

½ small fennel bulb

1 apple

2 carrots

¼ beetroot

Juice all ingredients in a juicer, and drink immediately.

* *

Raspberry Green Smoothie

(Makes 1 quart)

2 Bosc pears

1 handful of raspberries

4-5 leaves kale

2 cups water

Blend all ingredients in a blender until smooth.

* *

Mediterranean Soup

(Makes 1 quart)

1 cup spinach

1 stalk celery

1 teaspoon oregano

1 teaspoon thyme

½ red bell pepper

½ avocado

½ cucumber

½ jalapeño pepper

2 tablespoons lime juice

¾ cup water

Dulse leaves or flakes—optional

Blend all ingredients in a blender until smooth.

* *

* *

Raw Corn Salad

(Makes 2 to 3 servings)

4 ears fresh corn on the cob

4 stalks celery

1 red bell pepper

4–5 radishes

1 medium avocado

Juice of 1 lime

½ head romaine lettuce

1 cup arugula

Arrange romaine lettuce and arugula on two or three plates. Spoon corn salad into a teacup or small bowl and turn onto the lettuce.

* *

Sea Vegetable Wraps

½ head romaine lettuce

½ carrot, shredded

¼ cup fresh alfalfa or broccoli sprouts

2 sheets nori, cut into 1- by 3-inch strips

Place a spoonful of sauce (see recipe below) at the top of a lettuce leaf. Add a pinch of sprouts, shredded carrot, and a strip of nori. Fold the top of the leaf over, and roll the entire lettuce leaf up tightly.

For the Sauce:

2 tablespoons dulse flakes

1 tablespoon tahini

1 tablespoon chia seeds, soaked for fifteen minutes

2 tablespoons fresh lemon juice

3 tablespoons water

Blend all ingredients in a blender until smooth. Allow sauce to sit for fifteen minutes. Add more water if necessary. The sauce should be thick so that it will stay put in the wrap.

* *

DAY SEVEN

Every day we are engaged in a miracle which we don't even
recognize: a blue sky, white clouds, green leaves, the black,
curious eyes of a child—our own two eyes. All is a miracle.
—*Thich Nhat Hanh*

Each day is precious. Each moment is precious—an opportunity to awaken to the incredible beauty of our lives. As you release toxins and eat more lightly, perhaps each day of the cleanse will bring you closer to this realization.

The gentle clearing out that you are experiencing during this first week of your cleanse is likely to bring greater clarity of mind. As you take away some of the things that slow you down on your path to physical health, you inevitably find that your way becomes clearer emotionally, mentally, and spiritually as well. The cleanse provides an opportune time to embark on the practice of mindfulness.

Mindfulness is the energy of being aware and awake to the
present. It is the continuous practice of touching life deeply in
every moment.
—*Thich Nhat Hanh*

There are many mindfulness practices that can help you to grow in awareness and be more fully present. As mentioned previously, the *breath* can be a powerful vehicle, bringing you into the here and now in a matter of a few seconds. You can incorporate simple breathing techniques into your day as often as you like. *Meditation* is also an extremely effective mindfulness practice. When you turn inward and heighten your perceptions, you cannot help but grow in awareness and self-understanding. Please try to find at least five minutes each day to be quiet and still and completely present.

I suggest that you carve out that time first thing in the morning. You will find that five minutes of meditation is far more valuable than five more minutes of sleep. It is too likely that other things will crowd out your meditation time if you leave it for later in the day. If you are interested in doing more meditation, it is better to increase the frequency rather than the length of your sessions. Instead of elongating each meditation session, do several five-minute meditation sessions scattered throughout the day. Not only will you be more alert and effective during the shorter meditations, you also will be allowing the practice of meditation to bring silence and tranquility to more parts of your day.

Another wonderful way to develop awareness is through the practice of *mindful eating*. Eating can be a meditative practice if we choose to make it such. As we serve our food, we realize that "many elements, such as the rain, sunshine, earth, and the care taken by the farmers and the cooks, have all come together to form this meal. In fact, through this food we see that the entire universe is supporting our existence. Food reveals our connection with the earth . . . the extent to which our food reveals itself depends on us. . . . Contemplating your food for a few seconds before eating, and eating in mindfulness, can bring you much happiness" (Thich Nhat Hanh).

Exercise for Day Seven

MANTRAS OR MINDFULNESS VERSES

One way to dwell in the present moment is to practice with phrases or mantras. Repetition of a mantra can deepen our experience of simple daily acts that we often take for granted. For today, you may want to try the mindfulness verse or mantra below.

When you turn on the water faucet, look deeply and see how precious the water is. There are so many people in the world who do not have enough to drink. Each time you turn on the water faucet today, think of this mantra, borrowed from Thich Nhat Hanh:

Water flows from high mountains.
Water flows from deep earth.
Miraculously water comes to us and sustains all life.

Every day we are engaged in a miracle. Each day is indeed precious, and we want to help ourselves to be awake and alive to all of it.

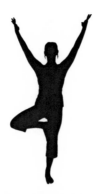

Yoga Pose for Day Seven
TREE POSE (*VRKSASANA*)

Benefits: Strengthens the muscles of the supporting foot and leg, helps to develop balance and concentration, and calms the mind.

Do not do this pose if you are feeling dizzy. Stand on your mat with your feet hip width apart. Shift your weight onto your left foot. Bend your right knee, and turn it out to the side. Place the sole of your right foot either on your left inner shin or on your left inner thigh. Reach down to position the foot if necessary. If the right foot is on the thigh, the foot should be at the middle of the thigh with the toes pointing downward and the bent right knee turned out to the side.

Maintain a gentle focus on a point out in front of you. As you inhale, you may stretch your arms up and overhead with your elbows straight. Hold the pose for five to ten breaths, coming out when you feel ready. Repeat the Tree Pose on the opposite side.

ESSENTIAL OILS

You may find it helpful during this cleanse to use some aromatherapy to promote relaxation and healing. In addition to addressing some of the symptoms that you may experience during the cleanse, in general, the use of essential oils also can be a welcome addition to a more mindful lifestyle because the scents can alter your mood in subtle yet powerful ways.

Essential oils are aromatic liquids derived from flowers, trees, shrubs, bushes, roots, and seeds. These oils defend plants from insects, the environment, and disease. They are also critical for a plant's growth and adaptation to its surroundings. Referred to as the *essence* of the plant, pure essential oils not only protect the plant but also determine its aroma.

Essential oils have been used in daily life for centuries as perfumes, in cooking, and for medicinal purposes. Inhaling essential oils heightens the senses and can trigger various responses in the body. Below are several methods for using essential oils:

❖ Direct inhalation—simply smell them.

❖ Diffuse the oils into a vapor using a diffuser.

❖ Add a few drops of oil to a bowl or pot of hot water. Cover your head with a towel, and breathe the vapor in slowly.

Combine the essential oil with vegetable oil such as almond oil or olive oil to avoid skin reactions. Apply this combination to

❖ The crown of the head

❖ The forehead

❖ The temples

❖ Behind the ears

❖ The neck or upper back

❖ The abdomen

❖ The soles and tops of the feet

❖ The ankles

Angelica root . . . *Detoxifies* • Arthritis, gout, nervous exhaustion. Do not use if pregnant or in direct sunlight, and do not use in a concentration of more than 1 percent.

Aniseed . . . *Antispasmodic* • For indigestion, flatulence, digestive problems, and spasms.

Basil, sweet . . . *Relieves mental fatigue* • Clears the head, gives strength and clarity, relieves migraines.

Bay leaf, wild . . . *Cough suppressant, scalp stimulant* • Clears dandruff, oily hair; promotes hair growth; relieves cough. Use in moderation, 1 percent or less in a blend.

Benzoin-absolute . . . *Expectorant* • Powerful healing effects on rashes, eczema, and dry and chapped skin. Helps to relieve nervous tension.

Bergamot . . . *Relieves anxiety* • Very uplifting and refreshing; reduces depression. Excellent for acne and stress-related eczema. Do not use in direct sunlight.

Bergamot-bergapten free . . . *Relieves anxiety* • Very uplifting and refreshing; reduces depression. Excellent for acne and stress-related eczema.

Birch, sweet wild . . . *Anti-inflammatory* • Good for arthritis; increases circulation; detoxifies. Harmful in high concentration; use less than 1 percent in a blend.

Carrot seed . . . *Treats skin problems* • Eczema, rosacea; revitalizes and tones mature and dry skin; helps to prevent and reduce wrinkles.

Cassia bark . . . *Antibacterial* • Use as an air deodorizer; antifungal and antiviral. Very irritating to skin. Avoid using during pregnancy or on children.

Cedarwood, Virginia wild . . . *Astringent* • Acne, oily skin and scalp, dandruff, hair loss, and psoriasis. Great insect repellent and room deodorizer. Avoid use during pregnancy.

Chamomile, blue . . . *Anti-inflammatory* • Soothes skin irritations; relieves headaches, migraines, insomnia, and inflamed joints and wounds. A nervous sedative.

Chamomile, Roman . . . *Analgesic* • Muscle and joint pain, eczema, headaches, migraines, and insomnia. Reduces nervous tension and depression. Very sedative. *Note:* Best chamomile for children.

Citronella . . . *Deodorizer* • Use as an insect repellent or a room deodorizer; very bactericidal. May cause dermatitis. Avoid using during pregnancy.

Clary sage . . . *Antispasmodic* • Female hormonal balancer; excellent for menstrual cramps and premenstrual syndrome (PMS). Avoid alcohol, and avoid use during pregnancy.

Clove bud . . . *Bactericidal* • Infections, athlete's foot, sprains, and toothaches. Use as a room freshener to deodorize. Repels insects and prevents colds. May cause skin irritations.

Coriander seed . . . *Analgesic* • Muscular aches and pains, poor circulation, stiffness and arthritis. Helps with mental fatigue, migraines, and exhaustion.

Cypress . . . *Antispasmodic* • Cellulite, muscular cramps, and varicose veins. Helps with asthma, bronchitis, and whooping cough.

Dillweed . . . *Digestion* • Great for colicky children as a massage; use only three drops per ounce of carrier. Relieves dyspepsia, flatulence, and indigestion.

Elemi, wild . . . *Antiseptic* • Prevents infection of cuts and wounds, inflammation, wrinkles, and dry skin; also used for bronchitis and coughs.

Eucalyptus globulus . . . *Expectorant* • Antiseptic; respiratory conditions—asthma, colds, and flu. Helps to regenerate lung tissue; helps to increase oxygen supply. Quite strong for children.

Eucalyptus radiata . . . *Anti-inflammatory* • Respiratory conditions, bronchitis, colds, and flu; great for asthma, muscular aches and pains, poor circulation, and sprains. Fine for use on children.

Fennel, sweet . . . *Digestion* • Abdominal cramping, flatulence, colic, constipation, glandular system, loss of appetite, nausea. Avoid use during pregnancy or if epileptic.

Frankincense . . . *Skin care* • Treats aging and dry skin, acne and scars, anxiety, and stress-related conditions; slows and deepens breathing; good for meditation. Avoid use during pregnancy.

Geranium . . . *Hormonal balancing* • Helps to regulate hormonal system; regenerates skin cells; good for eczema, scars, nervous tension, and depression.

Ginger root . . . *Analgesic* • Indigestion, nausea, diarrhea. Relieves arthritis and rheumatism; very warming to the muscular system. Do not use in direct sunlight.

Grapefruit . . . *Stimulant* • Acne, oily skin; promotes hair growth and reduces muscle fatigue. Relieves cellulitis and water retention; helps to reduce depression.

Helichrysum . . . *Healing* • Abscesses, acne, boils, burns, cuts, eczema, inflammation, severe scars, and wounds; relieves aches and pains and strained muscles.

Hyssop, wild . . . *Antispasmodic* • Asthma, bronchitis, tonsillitis, indigestion, colds, flu, and whooping cough. Avoid if pregnant or epileptic. Do not use in high doses.

Jasmine . . . *Intoxicating* • Stimulates the brain to release encephaline, a neurotransmitter that acts as an antidepressant and aphrodisiac. Avoid use during pregnancy.

Juniper berry . . . *Detoxify* • Releases accumulated fluids and toxins; treats cellulitis, gout, and rheumatism. Avoid use during pregnancy or if you have kidney disease.

Lavender . . . *Balancing (most versatile oil)* • Burns, eczema, insomnia, headaches, infections, flu, wounds, and muscular aches; calms and relaxes.

Lemon . . . *Astringent* • Acne, boils, oily skin, and herpes infections; aids in the removal of cellulite. Refreshing; clears the mind. Do not use in direct sunlight.

Lemongrass . . . *Antiseptic* • Purifier and room deodorizer, disinfectant, insect repellent; infectious diseases, excessive perspiration, acne, and athlete's foot.

Lime . . . *Lymphatic stimulant* • Water retention, gall bladder and liver congestion, cellulitis; increases circulation; refreshing and uplifting. Do not use in direct sunlight.

Litsea cubeba, wild . . . *Digestion* • Flatulence and indigestion; very antiseptic; relieves acne, excessive perspiration, and greasy skin; good insect repellent.

Mandarin . . . *Refreshing* • Great for children; helps them sleep. Prevents stretch marks and scarring. Use only one to five drops per ounce of unscented carrier.

Marjoram, sweet . . . *Analgesic* • Antiviral, bactericidal, relieves PMS, sprains, and bronchitis; relieves nervous tension, migraines, and headaches. Avoid use during pregnancy.

Myrrh . . . *Skin conditions* • Athlete's foot, dry mature skin, scars, eczema, hemorrhoids, and thrush. Also quite sedative; great for meditation. Avoid use during pregnancy.

Myrtle, red . . . *Antiseptic* • Astringent, bactericidal, expectorant; relieves bronchitis, tuberculosis, colds, flu, infectious disease, acne, open pores, and hemorrhoids.

Neroli . . . *Stress* • Helps anxiety, depression, shock; lowers brain activity; relaxes and calms the spirit.

Niaouli, wild . . . *Antispasmodic* • Respiratory problems, allergies, and asthma; great for bronchitis. Use as a room deodorizer to relieve coughs, sinusitis, colds, and flu.

Nutmeg . . . *Analgesic* • Arthritis, gout, poor circulation, indigestion; can reduce frigidity and impotence. Use in small doses only; sedative effects. Avoid use during pregnancy.

Orange, sweet . . . *Antidepressant* • Refreshing; clears the mind of worry and negativity; very calming, helps to stop hysteria, and combats insomnia. Excellent as a room freshener. Do not use in direct sunlight.

Oregano . . . *Bactericidal* • Use as a room deodorizer to prevent infection and the spread of viruses. *Warning:* Skin irritant. Avoid use during pregnancy.

Palmarosa . . . *Antiseptic* • Cell regeneration, acne, minor skin infections; regulates sebum production, oily/dehydrated skin, and scars. Relieves nervous exhaustion and stress-related conditions.

Parsley seed . . . *Diuretic* • Accumulation of toxins, broken blood vessels, and cellulitis. Also aids in digestion, hemorrhoids, and flatulence. Avoid use during pregnancy.

Patchouli . . . *Skin healing* • Tissue regenerator, wrinkles, and weeping eczema. Helps to close pores and kill bacteria. Very calming, grounding; good for frigidity.

Pepper, black . . . *Stimulant.* Digestive problems—constipation, diarrhea, flatulence, heartburn, loss of appetite, and nausea. Also used as an aphrodisiac.

Peppermint . . . *Stimulant* • Very cooling and anti-inflammatory to muscles; reduces swelling, pain and bruising, migraines, and nausea. A mental stimulant. Avoid use during pregnancy.

Peru balsam . . . *Skin problems* • Dry and chapped skin, eczema. Helps to relieve asthma, bronchitis, and coughs. Like other balsams, has a warming and comforting quality.

Petitgrain . . . *Stress* • Mental fatigue and strain. For stress, anxiety, and depression. Increases concentration, and clears mind of worry and obsessive thoughts.

Pine needles . . . *Expectorant* • Sinus and respiratory problems, asthma, infection; stimulates adrenal glands. A great air antiseptic, refreshes, cleanses, and soothes the mind.

Rose Otto . . . *Well-being* • The rose gives one thing above all: happiness. Helps with managing grief, depression, and emotional shock.

Rosemary . . . *Fatigue* • Intellectual strain, poor memory and concentration; good for hair care. Do not use if epileptic. Avoid use during pregnancy.

Rosewood, wild . . . *Antiseptic* • Skin care—cellular stimulant, dry mature skin, ear infections (rub around the ear, not in it), wrinkles, and scars. Also calming and good for anxiety and sadness.

Sage . . . *Cleansing* • Used by Native Americans for ceremonial cleansing of their homes. Stops cramping during menstruation. Avoid use during pregnancy.

Sandalwood . . . *Grounding* • Centering; helps with depression and anxiety; corresponds to male pheromone; helps with meditation.

Spearmint . . . *Stimulant* • Very cooling and anti-inflammatory to muscles; reduces swelling, pain, bruising, migraines, and nausea. A mental stimulant. Avoid use during pregnancy.

Tea tree . . . *Antiviral, antifungal* • Acne, sinus and respiratory congestion, vaginitis, herpes, and parasites; immune stimulant; safely applicable to skin; anti-inflammatory.

Thyme . . . *Bactericidal.* • Acne, cuts, insect bites, lice, gum infections, oily skin, and scabies. Avoid use if pregnant or have high blood pressure.

Valerian root . . . *Calming* • Good for insomnia; hypnotic and sedative. Relieves nervousness, indigestion, and migraines. Helps restlessness and tension.

Vetiver, root . . . *Relaxing* • Deeply relaxing for anyone experiencing stress and depression; has sedative effects and is great for insomnia. Also relieves arthritis and muscular aches.

Ylang-ylang . . . *Aphrodisiac* • Helps to reduce high blood pressure and heart palpitations. Calming; relieves insomnia and depression. Soothes and inhibits anger born of frustration.

RECIPES FOR DAY SEVEN

* *

Mixed Vegetable Juice

1 kale leaf

1 collard leaf

Small handful of parsley

1 stalk celery

1 carrot, greens removed

½ red pepper

1 tomato

1 broccoli floret

Celery stalk for garnish

Juice leaves and parsley and then the celery and carrot. Follow with red pepper, tomato, and broccoli. Garnish with celery stalk.

* *

Berry-Banana Smoothie

2 cups fresh blueberries, raspberries, strawberries

1 banana

1 orange

Blend all ingredients in a blender until smooth.

* *

Lemon-Mint Soup

2 apples

½ lemon

2 cups mesclun or spring salad mix

2 tablespoons Bragg's liquid aminos

1 avocado

1 cup fresh mint

4 cups water

Blend ingredients in a blender until creamy.

* *

Refreshing Summer Salad

(Makes 1 to 2 servings)

1 cup fresh arugula or spinach

1 avocado, sliced

1 bulb fennel, julienned

½ cup sweet cherry or grape tomatoes, halved

1 orange bell pepper, julienned

¼ cup sliced scallions

1 tablespoon fresh dill—optional

¼ cup fresh lemon juice

Liquid stevia, several drops to taste

Combine all the vegetables, and toss together.

Raw Chili

1 zucchini, chopped into ½-inch cubes

1 carrot, chopped into ¼-inch cubes

½ small eggplant, peeled and chopped into ½-inch cubes

1 small Portobello mushroom or 5 shiitake mushrooms, chopped into cubes

3 cloves garlic, crushed

1 medium Roma tomato, chopped into ½-inch cubes

¼ medium red onion, chopped

3½ teaspoons sea salt

1 tablespoon lemon juice

2 tablespoons extra-virgin olive oil

Mix all ingredients together and place in a quart-sized jar. Press down firmly so that the vegetables are completely immersed in the salt, lemon, and oil. Cover and let marinate for at least four to six hours or overnight.

For the Chili Sauce:

1 large tomato

1 cup sun-dried tomatoes, soaked with enough water to cover

¼ cup olive oil

1½ cups purified water

⅛ teaspoon cayenne pepper

½ tablespoon celery seed

½ tablespoon oregano

½ teaspoon cumin

1½ teaspoon chili powder

Blend ingredients on high until smooth. Pour blended mixture over marinated vegetables or pulse together in food processor.

DAY EIGHT

It's not how much we give but how much love we put into giving.

—Mother Teresa

When we bring mindfulness to the ordinary moments of our day, we find opportunities to make some of our activities an offering to others. Simply by being more fully present and attentive to our tasks and setting the intention to offer our efforts for the people we care about, our everyday activities gain beauty and meaning.

Exercise for Day Eight

KITCHEN MEDITATION

We can choose to be mindful when we are preparing our food, thus transforming our kitchen into a meditation room.

You might consider placing some small token—a beautiful stone, a simple leaf or twig, or a small flower vase—in a special spot in your kitchen. When you enter your kitchen, practice a few moments of conscious breathing. Then do your tasks in a calm, relaxed way. Bring gentle attention to your work, and infuse the healthy food you prepare with love. I like the "kissing the pan" tradition: Whenever you prepare a dish that will be shared with others, you can "kiss the pan" and make a wish that everyone who partakes also will take in the love and well wishes that you impart. This will be a gift to yourself and to those you serve.

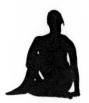

Yoga Pose for Day Eight

SEATED SPINAL TWIST
(*MODIFIED ARDHA MATSYENDRASANA*)

Benefits: Increases flexibility of the spine, improves breathing
by opening the chest and the muscles that support the rib
cage, and stimulates the digestive system.

Do not practice this pose if you have diagnosed disk disease in your lower back. If you are pregnant, come into the twist gently, and let your belly stay soft. Sit in a comfortable, cross-legged seat. Lift your right knee, and place your right foot on the floor just outside your left knee. Make your right hip heavy, weighting it firmly into the floor. Gently twist your torso to the right, bringing your right fingertips to the floor behind your tailbone. Wrap your left elbow around your right knee, and hug your right knee into your chest as you lift up through your spine. Glance over your right shoulder as you draw the shoulder back, and create a deeper twist for the spine. Take three to five deep breaths in this Seated Spinal Twist Pose before releasing. You may do this twist two to three times on each side.

For some of you, cutting out meat, poultry, fish, eggs, and dairy will be a radical departure. Even if you are just eliminating animal protein for a few weeks, you still may be concerned about not getting adequate protein. How much protein do you really need, and does a vegan diet meet the mark? Health organizations typically cite an optimal protein requirement of around 10 percent of total calories. The recommended daily allowance (RDA) on food packages also lists daily protein requirements at 10 percent.

While Americans average around 15 to 16 percent of calories from protein, most experts agree that only 5 to 6 percent of dietary protein is required to replace the protein regularly excreted by the body in the form of amino acids. When protein rises above 10 percent of calories, it begins to have a detrimental effect on health and can result in autoimmune disease, cancer, and impaired liver and kidney function.

Excess protein from animal sources is extremely acidifying. It causes the body to strip calcium from the bones in order to counteract the excessive acid. Moreover, animal protein is high in fat and cholesterol: Eggs are 60 percent fat, as is ground beef. Cheddar cheese is 72 percent fat.

If you are concerned that a vegan diet will not provide enough protein for the next few weeks, bear in mind that *all* plant foods contain protein. The following list provides a basis for comparison:

Protein source	Protein content
Beef	50%
Eggs	37%
Asparagus	36%
Sprouts	35%
Broccoli, frozen	34%
Spinach	30%
Peanuts	30%
Cauliflower	27%
Peas	27%
Whole milk	23%
Green leaf lettuce	22%
Green beans	18%
Bread, whole wheat	17%
Walnuts	17%
Spaghetti, whole wheat	16%
Macaroni, white	16%
Bread, white	14%
Cucumber	12%
Cantaloupe	11%
Celery	11%
Avocado	11%
Strawberry, fresh	8%
Rice, steamed	7%
Navel orange	7%
Carrots	6%
Watermelon	6%
Banana	5%
Raisins	4%
Peach	4%
Blueberry	3%
Pineapple	3%

If you eat a diet of 100 percent raw fruits and vegetables, protein probably will comprise about 5 percent of your calories. By adding a small amount of raw nuts and seeds, seed and/or nut milks, and nut butters, you will increase your protein intake a few percentage points, bringing you close to the recommended 10 percent. Moreover, you will be treating yourself to nutritious, fiber-filled foods, cleaning out your cells, and detoxifying your system.

On a vegan diet, you also want to be mindful about getting enough of the amino acid lysine. Legume-based foods, such as soybeans and their products (tempeh, tofu, soy milk, soy meats, etc.), beans (garbanzo, kidney, pinto, etc.) and their products (falafel, hummus, etc.), peas (green, split, and black-eyed), and lentils are good sources of lysine.

RECIPES FOR DAY EIGHT

Ginger Grape Juice

2 cups red grapes

2 inches fresh ginger, peeled

1 Meyer lemon, peeled

½ cup water, optional

Juice all ingredients in a juicer, and drink immediately.

Energizing Smoothie

(Makes 2 quarts)

2 cups green or red seedless grapes

3 golden kiwis, peeled

1 ripe orange, peeled, seeds removed

1 small leaf of aloe vera, with skin

5 leaves red leaf lettuce

2 cups water

Blend all ingredients together in a blender until smooth.

Raw Orange-Tomato Soup

3 tomatoes, diced

2 oranges, peeled and sliced

¼ cup sun-dried tomato slices, soaked for thirty minutes and drained

1 inch fresh ginger, peeled

Fresh basil leaves for garnish

Process all ingredients in a blender or food processor. Garnish with fresh basil leaf, and serve with a side of fresh sprouts.

Fennel Salad

1 large fennel bulb, shredded

1 red bell pepper, cut into two-inch-long thin strips

1 cucumber, diced

½ avocado, chopped

Juice of 1 lemon or lime

2 tablespoons hemp seeds

Toss all ingredients together in a bowl, and enjoy.

Mushroom Fettucini Alfredo

(Makes 3 to 5 servings)

5–6 medium zucchinis, peeled

With a vegetable peeler, slice thin strands of zucchini. Set aside.

For the Mushroom Sauce:

¾ cup soaked dried mushrooms or 1 cup fresh mushrooms

¾ cup soaked cashews

¾ to 1 cup water

1 tablespoon extra-virgin olive oil

1 tablespoon raw agave nectar

2 tablespoons fresh lemon juice

¼ teaspoon dried white pepper

Sea salt to taste

Process all ingredients for the mushroom sauce in a blender or food processor until smooth. Add the sauce to the pasta. Toss well, and let sit for half an hour before serving.

DAY NINE

To love deeply in one direction makes us more loving in all others.

—Anne-Sophie Swetchine

Setting out on a spiritual journey requires strength and courage. Staying on track requires love. Love is the fuel that keeps us moving onward and upward. We can use specific practices, such as yoga and meditation, to awaken and enliven our innate capacity for love.

We cannot accept others deeply unless we are able to receive the love that accepts us deeply. We begin by trying to look at ourselves through the eyes of understanding and compassion. The relationship we have with our own mind and body directly influences how we relate to others. This is one of the reasons yoga can be such a powerful tool for developing kindness and universal love. Yoga lets us start there—with our own minds and bodies—to cultivate self-acceptance and to let go of our critical attitudes toward ourselves. When we can love more deeply in that one direction, it makes us more loving in all other directions.

Today's exercise is a meditation on loving kindness. It involves the use of mantras—simple phrases that may be repeated—in order to cultivate particular qualities such as compassion, patience, generosity, and serenity. Today's mantras relate to self-understanding and are particularly powerful. It is helpful to repeat this exercise regularly for several days or weeks until the sense of loving kindness and acceptance toward yourself begins to grow.

Exercise for Day Nine

CULTIVATING LOVING KINDNESS

This meditation is a 2,500-year-old practice that uses repeated phrases or mantras to evoke and develop compassion or loving kindness (also called *metta*) toward oneself and others. In this particular practice, the focus is on the self as a starting point. Sit comfortably in a quiet place. Consciously relax. Begin to recite inwardly the following phrases, directed toward yourself: "May I be filled with loving kindness. May I be well. May I be peaceful and at ease. May I be happy."

Repeat these phrases over the course of five to ten minutes, perhaps holding an image in your mind of yourself as a child or as you are now. If possible, practice this loving-kindness meditation for five to ten minutes each day over several weeks.

Loving kindness is the soil from which our spiritual life can grow and flourish. If we can cultivate a loving heart, then all our encounters and experiences will flow more smoothly, and our compassion will be wide and expansive. I hope that today's message reminds you that you are worthy of love. May we see ourselves thus and learn to extend love in all directions.

You, more than anyone on this planet, deserve your love and affection.

—*The Buddha*

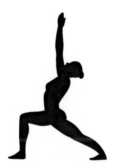

Yoga Pose for Day Nine

WARRIOR ONE (*VIRABHADRASANA ONE*)

Benefits: Strengthens the thighs, stretches the calf of the back leg, and increases flexibility in shoulders and upper back.

Stand on your mat with your feet about four to four and a half feet apart. Lift your arms out to the sides, and turn both feet to the right. Inhale as you stretch your arms long overhead. As you exhale, turn your torso to face your right leg. Press your left heel firmly into the floor, and engage the muscles of your left leg. Bend your right knee, ideally bringing your right thigh parallel to the floor. Draw your left hip forward as you also shift your left shoulder forward. You do not need to come all the way to a right angle with the right leg right away. This will come with practice. The main action of the pose is to square the hips and the shoulders. Hold the pose for several breaths, and change sides.

There is considerable confusion and debate about the value of dairy products. If they are currently a staple of your diet, perhaps you are wondering about doing without them for the next two weeks. For the purposes of this cleanse, it is helpful to remove dairy products from your diet so that the extra raw fruits and vegetables and fresh juices can be more effective cleansers. Since I am on the subject of dairy products, I thought I would provide some information here, simply food for thought about the relative value of dairy in our diet.

Cow's milk has three times more protein than human milk and a bit less fat. (In the case of the frequently recommended nonfat milk, it has *no* fat.) Human milk also has twice as many carbohydrates as cow's milk. Some believe that the ratio of these nutrients indicates that cow's milk is not designed for the human body. This high protein content, along with lactose intolerance, makes dairy the number one allergen by far. Some medical experts assert that when we consume foods that are not digested properly, especially those with anabolic (buildup) properties such as protein and calcium, the excess is not eliminated efficiently and leads to problems of excretion such as asthma, allergies, strep throat, tonsillitis, ear infections, acne, overweight, and excessive mucous and phlegm.

Lactose intolerance is extremely common. By the time we reach late childhood or adolescence, 70 percent of people have lost the enzyme required to break down lactose (milk sugar). It is less commonly known that many people are also allergic to the proteins in dairy: casein and whey.

Although it may sound counterintutive, the consumption of milk and dairy products in fact contributes largely to a deficiency of calcium in the body. Actually, countries that have the highest dairy intake also have the highest incidence of osteoporosis. There are several explanations for this:

1. Cow's milk has a lower ratio of calcium to phosphorous (1.27:1 versus 2.35:1 in human milk). Phosphorous binds to calcium in the digestive tract, making it less absorbable.
2. If you are unable to digest lactose, as most people are, it ferments in your digestive tract. This produces lactic acid, which binds with the calcium and magnesium, making them less available for the body.
3. Fifty percent of available calcium in milk is lost through the process of pasteurization.
4. Low-fat and skim milk lack the fat necessary for transport of calcium through cell walls.

That being said, the most common concern with regard to eliminating dairy products is that one will become deficient in calcium. A vegan diet does provide alternative sources of calcium. Most vegetables, especially green ones such as broccoli and dark leafy greens, provide between 20 and 75 milligrams of calcium per half cup. Nut and seed butters and milks are also excellent sources of calcium. Since these products are not heated or cooked, the calcium is highly absorbable.

The following table shows various calcium sources and the amounts of calcium they provide in a typical serving:

Cow's milk	1 cup	288 milligrams
Almonds	¼ cup	150 milligrams
Hazelnuts	¼ cup	106 milligrams

Sesame seeds	2 tablespoon	264 milligrams
Walnuts	¼ cup	54 milligrams
Sunflower seeds	¼ cup	65 milligrams
Wakame seaweed	½ cup	150 milligrams
Agar or kelp seaweed	½ cup	60 milligrams
Chickpeas	1 cup	80 milligrams
Navy beans	1 cup	128 milligrams
Soybeans	1 cup	460 milligrams
Tofu	1 cup	258 milligrams
Tempeh	1 cup	172 milligrams
Pinto beans	1 cup	82 milligrams
Blackstrap molasses	1 tbsp	137 milligrams

As you can see, it is not as difficult as you might believe to get calcium from non-dairy food sources. In addition, vegetarians require less calcium intake because the absence of animal foods in the diet makes calcium more absorbable.

There are also some practical ways to ensure that your body does not lose the calcium it does get:

❖ *Reduce your caffeine intake* (i.e., coffee, tea, soda, and chocolate). Caffeine causes increased calcium loss in urine.

❖ *Reduce your intake of refined sugar.* Sugar increases calcium loss in urine.

❖ *Reduce your phosphorous intake.* Soda is the biggest source of phosphorous in most people's diets. Cow dairy products and red meat also contain phosphorous, which binds to calcium and makes it less absorbable.

❖ *Reduce salt.* Salt increases calcium loss in urine.

❖ *Get your vitamin D.* Receive at least twenty minutes of sun exposure several times a week, or take vitamin D supplements. Calcium cannot be used by the body in the absence of vitamin D

❖ *Do not overeat protein.* Protein is acid forming; the body will protect the more alkaline pH level of the blood by pulling minerals (especially calcium) from the bones to buffer the acidity.

❖ *Reduce or eliminate nicotine, alcohol, and corticocosteroid medications.* These substances also contribute to calcium loss.

Your choice about whether to include dairy products in your diet going forward is entirely personal, and each individual's constitution will react differently. This cleanse provides you with an opportunity to see how you feel without dairy products and make a more informed decision about their role in your diet in the future.

RECIPES FOR DAY NINE

· ·

Apple-Celery Juice

1 stalk celery

2 apples

Juice all ingredients in a juicer, and drink immediately.

· ·

Watermelon-Spinach Smoothie

½ small seeded watermelon, including the peel

10 strawberries

1 bunch spinach

1 cup water

Blend all ingredients in a blender until smooth.

· ·

Raw Vegetable Delight Soup

(Makes 2 servings)

1 cup tomatoes, chopped

1 cloves garlic, minced

2 cups onion, chopped

1 cucumber, peeled and diced

1 yellow squash, chopped

1 zucchini, chopped

1 cup celery, diced

2 cups red bell pepper, diced

½ ear corn, kernels cut off cob

2 teaspoons sea salt

2 teaspoons dried dill or ½ teaspoon fresh dill

Blend all ingredients in a blender or food processor to desired consistency. Garnish with slices of cucumber and a sprinkle of fresh dill.

· ·

Summer Green Salad with Avocado and Cashew Tarragon Dressing

(Makes 2 to 4 servings)

3 cups greens, such as watercress, chard, and arugula

2 cups spinach

1 tablespoon fresh mint

½ cup baby tomatoes, cut into quarters

½ cucumber, diced

1 red pepper, sliced or diced

1 avocado, cut into a fan

1 tablespoon lemon juice

2 teaspoons olive oil

Combine greens, spinach, red pepper, and cucumber. Just before serving, toss the salad with the lemon juice and olive oil. Top with avocado.

For the Dressing:

½ cup cashews, soaked overnight

¼ cup water

2 tablespoons fresh tarragon

½ clove garlic

1 tablespoon apple cider vinegar

1 teaspoon lemon juice

3 tablespoons olive oil

Water as needed to blend

Blend all ingredients in a blender until smooth. Pour over salad when ready to serve.

* *

Spicy Raw Rice

1 small head cauliflower

¼ head green cabbage

½ hot pepper

½ bunch cilantro

Handful of chopped dulse

½ medium diakon radish

1 inch fresh ginger

Juice of 1 lemon or lime

2 tablespoons hemp seeds—optional

Process all the ingredients except the hemp seed in several batches in your food processor with the S-shaped blade until all the vegetables are the about the size of half grain of rice. Mix in the hemp seeds, and serve as a main course or a side dish.

* *

DAY
TEN

To undertake a genuine spiritual path is not to avoid difficulties
but to learn the art of making mistakes wakefully, to bring to
them the transformative power of our heart.

—*Jack Kornfield*

Congratulations. You are approaching the halfway point of this twenty-one-day cleanse. As you may have seen by now, cleansing physically can be a powerful catalyst, stirring up issues and emotions that tend to bring along with them some degree of discomfort and struggle. From a spiritual perspective, each of the inevitable difficulties we encounter can be a source of awakening. Our problems then become the very place where we discover wisdom and love.

As you prepare to enter the second half of your cleanse, you also need to prepare to meet the difficulties that might arise with a mindful, receptive attitude. You can begin by seeking to recognize and understand what you usually do when faced with either external challenges or your own limitations. What is your typical response? When we quiet ourselves in meditation, our process of reacting becomes clear. This makes meditation a potent means of self-discovery. Over the next few days, allow your personal difficulties and the issues you struggle with to enter into your meditation sessions, and watch what happens.

Exercise for Day Ten

WELCOMING YOUR DIFFICULTIES

Sit in a quiet place. Tune into your breathing. Allow yourself to become calm and receptive. Bring to mind a difficulty that you are facing in your spiritual practice or in any aspect of your life. As you focus on this difficulty, notice what happens in your body, heart, and mind.

Ask yourself a few questions. Listen to your inner voice for the answers.

How have I treated this difficulty so far?
Has my response brought me peace or more suffering?
What does this struggle or issue ask me to let go of?
What part of this difficulty is inevitable or unavoidable? How much of
   it do I need to simply accept?
What bigger lesson might this difficulty teach me?
What is the hidden value in this struggle?

Take your time with this reflection. Perhaps you will want to repeat it several times to allow the understanding and the opening to come slowly.

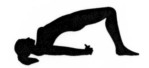

Yoga Pose for Day Ten
BRIDGE POSE
(*SETU BANDHA SARVANGASANA*)

Benefits: Strengthens the middle and lower back; strengthens the hamstrings, quadriceps, and the buttocks; and increases flexibility in the chest, abdomen, upper back, shoulders, and wrists. Especially helpful if you have been sitting for long periods.

Do not do this pose during the second or third trimesters of pregnancy or if you have a hiatal hernia. Lie on your back with your knees bent and the soles of your feet on the floor parallel to one another, hip width apart with the heels close to the buttocks. As you inhale, press down into your heels, and lift your hips up off the floor. Slide your arms under your back, and bring your hands together, interlacing your fingers with your arms straight. Be sure that your shins are perpendicular to the floor. Draw your tailbone toward the backs of your knees to lengthen the lower spine. Press your chest back toward your chin. Take several deep full breaths before moving the arms apart and bringing your pelvis down to the floor. You may repeat this Bridge Pose three to four times.

The change to a much lighter diet can cause some initial constipation or irregularity. This is the last thing you want during a cleanse. As the enzyme-rich, vital raw foods do their cleansing work and your cells release toxins, you need to eliminate the poisons that are flooding your system. You can begin with a few commonsense steps, such as drinking lots of fluids and eating plenty of fresh, juicy raw fruit. Limit your consumption of concentrated foods such as nuts and seeds and cooked grains because they will be more binding and inhibit elimination. Try to move your body every day—do some yoga, ride your bike, or take a walk or a light run. Practice mindful breathing for at least a few minutes each day. Do your best to relax. Our bodies work so much better if we can let go of tension and trust our natural rhythms.

I rcommend that you avoid the use of laxatives because they can be extremely harsh, and it is not helpful to use even the natural, herbal variety laxatives on a regular basis. Enemas can be useful in relieving occasional constipation. You may find their use particularly helpful during this cleanse if your elimination is sluggish. Colonic irrigation is extremely beneficial, provided that you work with an experienced therapist. If possible, I recommend that you schedule a colon hydrotherapy session at some point during the final week of the cleanse. It will be highly effective in removing the waste that is being released into your system as a result of the dietary changes.

RECIPES FOR DAY TEN

• •

Rejuvenating Juice

Handful of parsley

3 carrots

2 stalks celery

2 cloves garlic

Juice all ingredients in a juicer, and drink immediately.

• •

Wake-up Smoothie

(Makes 2 quarts)

½ bunch dandelion greens

2 stalks celery

½ inch fresh ginger root

2 peaches

½ pineapple

Blend all ingredients together in a blender until smooth.

• •

Celeriac and Green Apple Soup

(Makes 2 cups)

2 cups peeled, chopped celeriac (celery root)

½ cup chopped green apple plus ½ cup diced fine for garnish

1 cup raw macadamia nuts, soaked for one hour or more

1 cup water

1 tablespoon coconut butter

3 tablespoons extra-virgin olive oil

2 tablespoons fresh lemon juice

2 tablespoons minced chives

Fresh chopped parsley, thyme, or rosemary for garnish

Blend celeriac and green apple in a blender until smooth. Pass mixture through a sieve or strainer, and discard pulp. Pour the strained liquid back into the blender along with the macadamia nuts, water, coconut butter, olive oil, and lemon juice. Blend thoroughly. Strain once again if desired. Season with sea salt and freshly ground pepper to taste.

Avocado-Kale Salad

½ head kale

1 avocado

4–5 radishes, sliced

1 cucumber, sliced

¼ cup raw almonds

2 tablespoons lemon juice

Sea salt to taste

Nutritional yeast—optional

Combine kale and avocado. Add cucumbers, radishes, and almonds, and toss gently. Add lemon juice, sea salt, other spices. Toss and serve.

Beet Stacks with Parsley Pesto and Sweet Pepper–Fennel Cream

(Makes 2 to 3 servings)

3 medium beets, peeled and sliced very thin on a mandoline or with a sharp knife or vegetable peeler

1 tablespoon extra-virgin olive oil

Sea salt and freshly ground black pepper to taste

Toss the beets with the olive oil, and sprinkle with a bit of salt and pepper until the beets are evenly coated.

For the Parsley Pesto:

2 cloves garlic

1½ cups raw pumpkin seeds, soaked for four to six hours, drained and rinsed

1 cup parsley leaves, well packed

¾ cup extra-virgin olive oil

¾ teaspoon sea salt

Process the garlic in a food processor until finely chopped. Add the remaining ingredients, and process until well combined.

For the Cream Sauce:

1 sweet bell pepper

½ cup carrots, roughly chopped

¼ cup extra-virgin olive oil

1 clove garlic

½ teaspoon sea salt

¾ teaspoon dried fennel seed

Blend the bell pepper, carrot, olive oil, garlic, and salt in a blender until smooth. Add the fennel seed, and blend lightly until just combined.

For the Assembly:

For each stack, begin with one slice of beet. Top with 2 teaspoons of parsley pesto. Cover with another slice of beet. Top with 2 more teaspoons of pesto and then a third slice of beet. Place a small spoonful of the sweet pepper sauce on top of the third beet. You may want to build several stacks at a time.

DAY
ELEVEN

The roots of all goodness lie in the soil of appreciation for goodness.

—The Dalai Lama

I invite you to nurture a sense of appreciation today. At several points throughout the day, you might take a moment to focus on the positive things that you often overlook in life: perhaps your sense of sight or hearing or some other aspect of your physical health or the fact that you have food and shelter and clothing. It takes only a second or two to bring yourself into a state of gratitude. But the effects of that state of mind extend far beyond the time we spend reflecting. When we realize how truly fortunate we are, the splendid, rich quality of our lives spreads out before us. *Let gratitude open the door to the fullness of life.*

Exercise for Day Eleven

GROWING APPRECIATION

Sit comfortably in a quiet place. Leave your thoughts about the past and the future aside. Breathe calmly, and close your eyes.

Think of three simple things for which you are grateful. Consider what life would be like without those three things.

Allow a feeling of gratitude to fill your heart. Relax into this state of appreciation, and abide there for several minutes. Observe the effect that a sense of appreciation has on your emotional state.

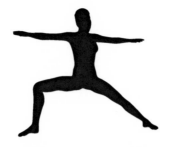

Yoga Pose for Day Eleven
WARRIOR TWO (*VIRABHADRASANA TWO*)

Benefits: Strengthens the hamstrings and quadriceps,
stretches the muscles in the pelvic region, and opens the hips.

Do not practice this pose if you have pain in your knee joints or if you are feeling unsteady or off balance. If you feel unstable, you may wish to do this pose with your back to a wall. Separate your feet four to four and a half feet apart (or one leg length apart), with your right toes pointing away from your body at a ninety-degree angle and your left toes turned in ten to fifteen degrees. Press firmly into the left foot, and engage the left leg. Bend the right knee while tracking the knee over the pinkie-toe side of the right foot. Draw the right side of the buttocks down and under. Reach your arms out to the side at shoulder height. Stretch back through your left arm so that the torso lines up directly over the hips. Turn your head to the right, and gaze out beyond your right fingertips. Hold this pose for three or four deep, steady breaths. Repeat several times on this side, and then change sides so that the left foot is in front and the left knee is bent. Repeat on the left side several times.

YOUR WORKPLACE

By now, most likely you have already found ways to adapt your daily routine to accommodate the cleanse. If you go to a workplace on a regular basis and are finding it difficult to maintain your intentions for the cleanse there, the following ideas may help:

- ❖ Bring a bag of fresh fruit to the office every day—bananas, grapes, berries, figs, apples. Be sure to include fruits that you truly enjoy eating.
- ❖ Double the recipe of your favorite raw salad dressing. Put half in your refrigerator at home and the other half in the fridge at the office. Bring your own salad to work, or use your raw dressing on a salad you purchase during your lunch break.
- ❖ Keep nuts, seeds, dried fruits, raw bars, and so on at your desk.
- ❖ Get out and walk during breaks and at lunchtime, even if it is just for a few minutes. Take that time to connect with your breath. Use your walks to slow down and bring yourself into the present moment.

❖ Practice simple breathing techniques throughout the day. Simply elongating the inhalations or exhalations will help you to stay connected to the here and now.

Eating with Friends

If you are uncomfortable about accepting invitations to eat with friends during this cleanse, consider that they actually may be inspired by the efforts you are making to care for yourself. There are many recipes to share, and you might be pleasantly surprised by how much a special homemade raw vegan dish will be appreciated by your friends. If you are eating out together, it will be quite easy to order a large salad or a fruit plate or other light vegetarian dish. Rather than feeling self-conscious and avoiding the company of friends or family, take this opportunity to share your journey and enjoy fresh, healthy food with people you care about.

On the Road

If you happen to be traveling for one or more days and are concerned about getting enough fresh, healthy cleanse-friendly foods along the way, simply plan to order raw salads and/or fruit plates when you eat out. Most restaurants will have some raw fruit or vegetables in the kitchen. You may be surprised by how accommodating most restaurants will be.

You also might consider bringing the following staples along with you on your trip:

lemons
apples
avocados
bananas

You also can bring the following items in dry form and then soak them overnight once you get to where you are staying:

prunes
dried figs
raw nuts and seeds
raw muesli (see recipe below)
dried seaweed (hijiki and arame are the best choices)

RECIPES FOR DAY ELEVEN

* *

Passion Juice

4 strawberries

½ pineapple

1 bunch black grapes

Juice all ingredients in a juicer, and drink immediately.

* *

Parsley Smoothie

(Makes 2 quarts)

1 bunch fresh parsley

1 cucumber, peeled

1 Fuji apple

1 ripe banana

1–2 cups water

Blend all ingredients together in a blender until smooth.

* *

Thai Soup

(Makes 1 serving)

1 cucumber

½ large avocado

1 lime, juiced

2 cloves garlic

3 leaves curly kale

¼ teaspoon tumeric powder

¼ inch fresh ginger root

1 cup water

Blend all ingredients in blender to desired consistency.

* *

* *

Asian Coleslaw

½ large napa cabbage, shredded

½ medium daikon radish, grated

1 cucumber, grated

½ bunch cilantro, chopped

⅓ cup wakame flakes, soaked for twenty to thirty minutes

1 avocado

Juice from 1 large lime

Mix all ingredients together and serve.

* *

Spicy Thai Vegetable Wraps

¼ cup raw cashews, chopped

2 teaspoons sesame oil

¼ teaspoon sea salt

2 tablespoons raw agave nectar

¼ cup lemon juice

1 tablespoon chopped ginger

2 teaspoons red chili pepper, seeds included, chopped

1 tablespoon Nama Shoyu soy sauce

1 cup raw almond butter

¼ head savoy cabbage, shredded

3 very large collard green leaves

½ large carrot, cut into matchstick-size pieces

½ large ripe mango, cut lengthwise into strips about ¼-inch thick

1 cup mung bean sprouts

¼ cup cilantro leaves

¼ cup basil leaves, torn

¼ cup mint leaves, torn or cut if leaves are large

For the Dipping Sauce:

3 tablespoons raw honey or raw agave nectar

1 tablespoon extra-virgin olive oil

Pinch of sea salt

Combine cashews, sesame oil, and sea salt, and set aside. Blend the honey or agave nectar, lemon juice, ginger, red chili pepper, and Nama Shoyu soy sauce in a blender until smooth. Add the almond butter, and blend at low speed to combine. Add water to thin, if necessary, to get a thick, cake batter–like consistency. Add this mixture to the shredded cabbage, and toss well to combine. Cut out the center rib of each collard green leaf, and divide the leaf in half. Place ½ leaf on a cutting board with the underside facing up. Arrange a few tablespoons of the cabbage mixture evenly across the bottom third of the leaf, leaving about 1½ inches clear at the bottom. Sprinkle some of the cashews over the cabbage. Lay a few sticks of carrot, a few strips of mango, and a few sprouts on top. Add several leaves each of cilantro, basil, and mint. Fold the bottom of the collard leaf up and over the filling, keeping it tight. Tuck the leaf under the ingredients, and roll forward. Place the roll seam side down on a serving dish. Repeat with remaining collard leaves and ingredients. Serve with the Dipping Sauce.

DAY TWELVE

Peace is every step.

—Thich Nhat Hanh

The first step of our spiritual journey is to realize that we have the potential to awaken. As we move along the path, we begin to recognize, define, and appreciate our authentic nature—our strongest potential for good. This potential often shows up for us in momentary flashes, but most of the time it is veiled in confusion, suffering, ignorance, fear, and anxiety. It is up to us to compile the spiritual tools we need to extract our purest qualities from the depths of our being, to uncover our innate purity, and to allow the full blossoming of our love.

Our practices of yoga and meditation are powerful tools. Use of the breath and the constant restating of our intentions keep us on track. The consistent effort to bring mindfulness to the present moment ensures that our journey is fruitful. We must remember that peace is every step.

If you do not have one already, now would be a good time to start a walking meditation practice.

We walk all the time, but often we are in a hurry, or we walk mindlessly, preoccupied with our plans or ruminating about something that has already happened. See if you can slow down and turn inward. As you walk, pay attention to each step you take. Become aware of how many steps you make with each breath, and then match your steps with your breath. When you breathe in, take two or three steps, depending on how long your in-breath takes. When you exhale, also count your steps. With practice, you will find that your inhalations and the exhalations even out, and it becomes easy to find a natural, relaxed rhythm.

You can practice walking meditation by counting your steps or by using words. *Peace Is Every Step* is the title of one of my favorite Thich Nhat Hanh books, and I have co-opted it as a kind of personal mantra. I have discovered that the phrase is perfectly suited to a walking meditation. I settle into a slow, steady walking pace. As I inhale, I say to myself, *"Peace is every step."* And with each exhalation, I repeat, *"Peace is every step."* You may want to try this out the next time you walk.

Exercise for Day Twelve

WALKING MEDITATION

Find a place—your driveway, the distance between two trees, a place in your yard, a stretch from the parking lot to your office—where you can walk quietly for just a few minutes. Five to ten minutes are enough.

Allow yourself to walk just for the sake of walking. The distance need not be far. In fact, it can be helpful to pace back and forth over a shorter distance rather than walking across a longer expanse. The pace should be slow. In this way, there is less of a sense of moving toward a destination and more of a sense of simply abiding in each step.

Concentrate intently on each step you take. Count the steps for each inhalation and for each exhalation. Continue counting or switch to marking the rhythm with such words as *"I am at peace"* or *"May I be at ease"* or *"Peace is every step"* or some other phrase that you like.

Peace is every step. The shining red sun is my heart. Peace is every step. It turns the endless path to joy.

—*Thich Nhat Hanh*

Yoga Pose for Day Twelve
CAMEL POSE (*USTRASANA*)
Benefits: Opens the chest, strengthens the muscles that line the spine, engages the quadriceps and buttocks, and creates greater range of motion in the thoracic (upper) spine.

Do not do this pose if you have high or low blood pressure, migraine headaches, or a serious low-back or neck injury. Kneel on your knees, with your knees hip width apart, thighs vertical, and shins parallel to one another, toes pointing straight back behind you. You may wish to fold your mat over or place a folded blanket under your knees for extra padding. Place your palms on your lower back with the fingertips pointing down. Bring your elbows toward one another, and lift your chest while pressing your hips forward. Remain in this gentle backbend or deepen the pose by first extending your right arm and reaching your right fingertips back to touch your right heel. Extend your left arm and bring your left fingertips to your left heel. Continue to lift the chest and press the hips forward. Hold for three to five deep breaths.

In addition to enhancing the cleansing process and promoting relaxation, the following self-care practices also let you focus on nurturing yourself. Rather than indulging in a heavier meal, it is often more supportive to take the time to care for your body in these alternative ways.

FOOT BATHS

Soaking your feet is a wonderful way to relax. You will need a basin that is large enough to place your feet in comfortably. Set aside ten to fifteen minutes to enjoy one of the following foot baths, perhaps in the evening after a long day.

These recipes have different effects. A salt foot bath relaxes the feet and takes away swelling. Essential oils are versatile: Lavender essential oil foot bath has a very relaxing effect, unlike the peppermint recipe, which rejuvenates the feet.

Baking Powder Foot Bath

Fill a large basin halfway with hot water, and add

- ❖ 3 tablespoons baking powder
- ❖ Several drops of tea tree oil
- ❖ ½ cup chopped parsley

Baking powder is an antibacterial agent that helps to prevent excessive perspiration and infections. Tea tree oil fights fungal infections and is an effective remedy for athlete's foot. Parsley is also antibacterial and improves circulation.

Salt Foot Bath

Fill a large basin halfway with hot water, and add

- ❖ ½ cup sea salt or Epsom salt

Salt relieves inflammation and soothes tired, achy feet.

Lavender Herbal Foot Bath

Fill a large basin halfway with hot water, and add

- ❖ 2 drops lavender essential oil
- ❖ 1 drop sandalwood or ylang-ylang oil—optional
- ❖ ¼ cup sea salt or Epsom salt

Lavender, sandalwood, and ylang-ylang each have a soothing effect.

Peppermint Foot Bath

Fill a large basin halfway with hot water, and add

- ❖ 3 drops peppermint essential oil
- ❖ 1 drop eucalyptus essential oil and 1 drop lemon essential oil

Peppermint, eucalyptus, and lemon oils have an invigorating effect and stimulate the circulation.

Softening Foot Bath

Fill a large basin halfway with hot water, and add

- ¼ cup fresh lemon juice
- 1 tablespoon cinnamon
- 2 tablespoons olive oil
- ¼ cup almond milk

This combination soothes and softens the skin.

NETI POT FOR NASAL IRRIGATION

The history of nasal cleansing began as an ancient ayurvedic technique in India. Originally used to clear the nostrils before yogic breathing, use of the neti pot has become part of regular self-care for many people with sinus and allergy issues. Rinsing the nasal passages with a saltwater solution helps to thin the mucus and clears the nostrils of irritants, allergens, and infectious agents. Irrigation also eases dry, irritated nasal passages, a common symptom in cold climates.

Dissolve one-quarter of a teaspoon of finely ground sea salt into eight ounces of water, and fill the neti pot with this solution. Stand over a sink or in the shower. Tilt your head to the side, bringing your ear toward your shoulder, and then tilt your head forward. Insert the spout of the neti pot into the upper nostril, and allow the water to flow into and through the nose. It should exit through the lower nostril. If water enters the back of your throat, increase the forward tilt of your head until the drip stops. After the rinse is finished, lean forward and allow any water to flow out. Blow your nose gently and thoroughly. Repeat the procedure on the other side. If your sinuses are inflamed or blocked, the water may not pass through the nostril initially. It might take a few tries for the water to flow freely through the sinus passages, but even the local irrigation provided by the water entering one nostril is helpful.

Please note that using a neti pot should not be painful. If you have a burning sensation or other type of pain in the nostrils during use, first check the water temperature. If the water that is too hot or too cold, this can cause discomfort. Next, assess the salt mixture. Too much or too little salt will create a burning sensation. If you are experiencing fever, severe headaches, bright green nasal discharge, or a productive cough, consult a physician or qualified health practitioner before using the neti pot. These can be signs of serious infection. Otherwise, the neti pot can be used daily.

CASTOR OIL PACKS

Castor oil packs are used by some alternative practitioners to stimulate circulation and to promote the healing of tissues and organs, to improve digestion, to enhance liver function, to relieve pain, and to reduce inflammation.

A castor oil pack can be placed on the following body regions:

- The right side of the abdomen (Some alternative practitioners recommend this as part of a liver detox program.)

❖ Inflamed and swollen joints, bursitis, and muscle strains

❖ The abdomen to relieve constipation and other digestive disorders

❖ The lower abdomen in cases of menstrual irregularities and uterine and ovarian cysts

To make a castor oil pack, you will need the following:

❖ Three layers of wool or cotton flannel large enough to cover the affected area

❖ Castor oil

❖ Plastic wrap cut one to two inches larger than the flannel (This can be cut from a plastic bag.)

❖ A hot-water bottle

❖ A container with lid

❖ Old clothes and sheets (Castor oil will stain clothing and bedding.)

Place the flannel in the container. Soak it in castor oil so that it is saturated but not dripping. Place the pack over the affected body part. Cover with plastic wrap. Place the hot-water bottle over the pack. Rest for forty-five minutes to an hour with the pack in place.

After removing the pack, cleanse the area with a solution of warm water and baking soda.

Store the pack in a covered container in the refrigerator. Each pack may be reused up to twenty-five to thirty times.

RECIPES FOR DAY TWELVE

Refreshing Ginger Fruit Juice

2 nectarines or peaches

½ cantaloupe

2 apples

1 inch fresh ginger claw

2 tablespoons ground flax seeds

Juice all ingredients in a juicer. Add 1 cup ice cubes, and blend in a blender until smooth.

Blueberry Smoothie

(Makes 1 quart)

1 stalk celery

2 cups fresh blueberries

1 banana

2 cups water

Blend all ingredients in blender until smooth.

Energy Soup

(Makes 2 servings)

2 medium beets, trimmed

2 medium carrots, trimmed

½ cucumber, peeled

½ cup avocado, mashed

⅓ cup cilantro leaves, loosely packed

3 cups water

2 tablespoons rice vinegar

1 tablespoon Nama Shoyu soy sauce or tamari

1 garlic clove, peeled and crushed

1 small chili pepper, stemmed and seeded

½ teaspoon cumin

1 cup corn, freshly cut off the cob

Grate the carrots, beets, and cucumber, and stir together in a bowl. Blend 3 cups of this grated mixture in a blender until smooth. Combine the blended mixture with the grated vegetables and the corn. Stir well and serve.

Mock Tuna Salad Using Juicer Pulp

Carrot or vegetable pulp from your juicer

Raw mayonnaise

Celery, diced

Onions, chopped

Spices to taste

Add raw mayonnaise (see recipe below) to your juicer pulp. Add other veggies to taste (e.g., scallions, celery, etc.). Add spices to taste.

For the Raw Mayonnaise:

½ cup soaked almonds or cashews

½ cup water (to desired consistency)

2 tablespoons lemon juice

½ clove garlic

½ tablespoon raw honey—optional

¼ teaspoon sea salt (or dried seaweed)

Raw apple cider vinegar to taste

Extra-virgin olive oil to taste

Blend all the ingredients except the olive oil in a blender until smooth. With blender still running, gradually add olive oil, and blend until emulsified.

Mushroom Fettucini Alfredo

(Makes 3 to 5 servings)

For the Fettucini:

5–6 yellow squash or zucchini

With a vegetable peeler, peel thin strands of the yellow squash or zucchini.

For the Mushroom Sauce:

¾ cup soaked dried mushrooms or 1 cup fresh mushrooms

¾ cup soaked raw cashews

¾–1 cup water

1 tablespoon extra-virgin olive oil

1 tablespoon raw agave nectar

2 tablespoons lemon juice

¼ teaspoon dried white pepper

Sea salt to taste

Process all ingredients in a food processor. Add the sauce to the squash or zucchini "pasta." Toss lightly, and allow to sit for half an hour before serving.

DAY THIRTEEN

If the person you are talking to doesn't appear to be listening, be patient. It may simply be that he has a small piece of fluff in his ear.

—*A. A. Milne,* Winnie-the-Pooh

In this final week of the cleanse, I hope that you are finding it easy and even fulfilling to eat a 100 percent raw diet of fruits and vegetables. If it is still feeling like a challenge to resist sugar, flour, animal products, or cooked food, please be gentle with yourself. If you get temporarily off track, you can always return to your intention and begin again.

A crucial part of the cleanse is learning to accept your humanness and approaching yourself with understanding and friendship. In driving ourselves to adhere to stringent guidelines in terms of what we eat or how we exercise, we can end up developing a subtle aggression against ourselves that completely defeats the overriding purpose of generating compassion. We need to listen attentively to our inner wisdom. If we are to grow in the direction of peace, deep listening is what is required.

Today, I suggest that you focus on this concept of deep listening. Through the practice of yoga, mindfulness meditation, and conscious breathing, you can develop a calm, quiet awareness that allows you to truly listen to yourself. Deep, attentive listening is also one of the best gifts we can give to another. Certainly, if we love someone, we will want to train ourselves to be better listeners. And perhaps if we do not feel that we love someone yet, our deep listening may open the door to love.

Exercise for Day Thirteen

DEEP LISTENING

Deep, attentive listening can be a meditation. Sit comfortably in a quiet place. Rest your awareness on your breath for several minutes. Then tune into your thoughts. Listen carefully to what they are saying.

Throughout your day, whenever someone is speaking to you, take a few deep, conscious breaths, and focus your full attention on listening calmly to the other's words. Notice if your mind is racing ahead to what you would like to say in response. Bring your attention back to the person who is speaking.

We learn so much from one another. Our spoken and unspoken words speak volumes about our fears, our hopes, our love. Let us listen carefully.

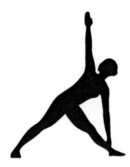

Yoga Pose for Day Thirteen
TRIANGLE POSE (*TRIKONASANA*)

Benefits: Strengthens the quadriceps, lengthens the hamstrings, opens the chest, strengthens the core muscles, stretches the spine, and improves balance.

Do not do this pose if it creates low-back pain. If you feel unsteady, you may practice this pose with your back against a wall. Stand with your feet at least one leg length apart, usually about four to four and a half feet apart. Turn your right toes away from the body at a ninety-degree angle, and be sure that the right kneecap is turning toward your right pinkie toe. Do not allow the kneecap to turn inward because this will strain the knee joint unduly. Turn the left toes inward ten to fifteen degrees. With both legs straight, press into your heels and lift your kneecaps to engage the leg muscles. Lift your arms out to the sides at shoulder height. Reach out with your right hand, bringing your right fingertips out beyond your right toes. Let your right hand fall to your right shin or higher. Stretch your left arm straight up toward the ceiling so that your left wrist lines up directly above your left shoulder. Contract the thighs, and expand across the chest. Take five to eight deep breaths. Repeat on the other side.

SEA VEGETABLES

Did you know that sea vegetables are twelve times more nutritious than the average vegetable? Seaweed is often referred to as an "ancient superfood." For thousands of years, our forefathers ate seaweed for optimal nutrition, and it has been considered a perfect food in China for over 2,000 years. Seaweed draws an extraordinary wealth of mineral elements from the sea that can account for up to 36 percent of its dry mass. Seaweed is high in iodine, calcium, magnesium, iron, vitamins C and A, protein, vitamins B_6 and B_{12}, fiber, alpha-linoleic acid, and omega-2 fatty acids, and in fact, seaweed contains more vitamins than fruits and vegetables. Raw or sun-dried seaweed contains

- High protein content—from 20 percent in green algae to 70 percent in spirulina
- High mineral content—especially iodine, calcium, iron, and magnesium
- More vitamin C than oranges
- Antiviral, antibacterial, and anti-inflammatory properties
- A large proportion of natural, organic iodine—which aids in maintaining healthy thyroid function
- A rich supply of calcium—much more than other plant sources
- Polysaccharides—important in the prevention of degenerative diseases, including cardiovascular disease and type 2 diabetes, in increasing the amount of "feel good" chemicals in the brain, in improving liver function, and in stabilizing blood sugar

Adding seaweed to your diet has the following health benefits:

- Healthy hearing
- Improved eyesight
- Clear skin
- Improved memory
- Healthy thyroid function
- Improved dental health
- Prevention of allergies and infections
- Lower blood pressure
- Healthier heart vessels
- Normalized cholesterol
- Overall improved digestion and waste elimination
- Increased level of "feel good" chemicals in the brain
- Improved liver function
- Stable blood sugar

You can buy sea vegetables in dried form at most health food stores. To use them, simply soak sea vegetables in water until soft. This usually takes only a few minutes. You also may reserve the nutritious soak water for use in soups or dressings.

Following is a list of commonly available and highly nutritious sea vegetables:

arame—a black seaweed that looks like angel hair pasta. It is wonderful tossed in salads or served on its own with chopped or shredded vegetables.

dulse—a burgundy-colored seaweed that can be eaten straight from the bag. It tears off in layers and melts in your mouth. You can keep fresh dulse moist and chewy by storing it in a sealed container. If it becomes dry and hard, soak it for a few minutes, drain, chop it up well, and add it to green salads. Use the soak water and/or the dulse itself in salad dressings. Dulse also mixes well with nuts as a snack. Dulse is often sold in powdered form, frequently combined with cayenne pepper or dried ginger. Powdered dulse is an excellent seasoning for salads, soups, or over an avocado.

kelp—a tough, thick seaweed usually sold in powdered form and used as a condiment. Kelp is the most nutritious of the seaweed varieties and perhaps the easiest to use.

kombu—Kombu resembles lasagne noodles and is often used in soups. It needs to be soaked for several hours until soft.

hijiki—Hijiki looks like black spaghetti. You need to soak it for at least an hour until it is completely soft. Drain well, and add to chopped or shredded vegetables.

RECIPES FOR DAY THIRTEEN

Sparkling Tropical Fruit Juice

1 kiwi, peeled
1 orange, peeled and sectioned
½ mango, peeled and sliced
Sparkling mineral water
Juice all ingredients in a juicer, and drink immediately.

Kale Smoothie

(Makes 1 quart)

5 leaves kale
¼ avocado
3 cloves garlic
Juice of ½ lime
2 cups water
Sea salt to taste
2 Roma tomatoes
Blend all ingredients in blender until smooth.

Raw Corn Chowder

2 ears fresh corn, kernels removed from cob

3 medium tomatoes, chopped

1 red bell pepper, chopped

1 cucumber

½ cup rough-cut okra

Handful of fresh basil leaves

Juice of ½ lemon

Small handful of dulse—optional

½ avocado

Process cucumber, tomato, okra, basil, dulse, and lemon juice in a food processor, and pulse until blended but still chunky. Add bell pepper, corn, and avocado, and blend to desired consistency. I prefer it with some texture and chunkiness to it.

Seaweed Salad

½ cup dried hijiki seaweed, soak in water for ten to twenty minutes or until softened, rinse, drain, and chop

1 apple, diced

1 cup cucumber, sliced thinly into quarter-moons

½ cup grated carrots

1 teaspoon freshly grated ginger or to taste

2 tablespoons sesame oil to taste

1 tablespoon apple cider vinegar

1 tablespoon Nama Shoyu soy sauce or tamari

1 clove garlic, minced

2 tablespoons sesame seeds

Combine all ingredients, and toss well.

Stuffed Red Peppers

(Makes 2 to 4 servings)

2 red bell peppers, cut in half with seeds/core removed

For the Filling:

1 cup soaked sunflower seeds

½ pint cherry tomatoes

1 stalk celery

½ teaspoon each of cayenne pepper, paprika, basil, oregano, and garlic

½ small onion, chopped

2 tablespoons lemon juice

1 tablespoon olive oil

Sea salt to taste

Process all ingredients in a food processor until thick and smooth.

For the Assembly:

Spoon about 2 tablespoons of the filling into each pepper half, and garnish with a parsley leaf.

DAY FOURTEEN

"When we accept what is in this very moment, without pushing or pulling, when there is no running after or running away, we find . . . a level of deep acceptance and peace."
—*Michael Stone*

Today's theme is to *slow down*. We spend so much of our lives running, and sometimes we move so fast that we miss the point. The experience we need most is the experience we are having at this moment. If we are rushing on to the next thing, we miss the experience—and the moment is gone. We cannot allow our lives to be a series of missed moments. Today, as much as possible, *try to slow down*.

Instead of racing home from work, encourage yourself to drive a little slower. If you usually jump out of bed and into the shower, perhaps you might add several steps in between: some gentle stretches, a few deep breaths, a look out the window.

If you are able to carve out a few minutes, it would be wonderful to spend time in a place of beauty: a garden, a park, in front of a favorite painting. You do not need to "do" anything—simply observe the beauty before you.

And most important, slow down long enough to truly see and hear the people in your life. Stop, look, and listen to others—your family, your friends, even the people you do not know well. They are your teachers; you need to show up for the lessons they offer. Slowing down makes you available to your experience moment by moment, as it unfolds. Give yourself that gift today.

Exercise for Day Fourteen

JUST SIT THERE

Take five minutes simply to sit in a quiet place with nothing to do. Close your eyes. Notice that initially your mind will want to go in a thousand directions. Just watch. Simply breathe. Slow down.

Rather than saying, "Don't just sit there, *do* something," instead, tell yourself, "Don' t *do* something, just sit there."

Yoga Pose for Day Fourteen
LOTUS POSE (*PADMASANA*)
Benefits: Calms the mind and allows for a deeper inner focus.
Stretches the front of the thighs, lengthens the spine, and
engages the core strength.

Sit in a comfortable cross-legged seat. In the full expression of Lotus Pose the feet rest on top of the thighs but this requires a high degree of flexibility in both the hip joints and the knee joints. If you are just beginning to explore Lotus Pose, simply allow the feet to be crossed loosely in front of you. You may want to sit on a folded blanket in order to lift your hips and relieve pressure in your knees, hips, and spine. Place your palms on your thighs, or let your hands fall loosely into your lap. You may also like to bring your palms to meet at the center of your chest in prayer position. Close your eyes, and take several long, deep breaths here. You may choose to take this time to do a brief meditation. Simply watch your breath for several minutes and observe your physical sensations as well as the thoughts that may arise.

BATHING

Bathing opens the pores and pulls waste-laden sweat out of your system, promoting the function of the skin as an organ of elimination and reviving the skin's youthful color and texture. More important, taking a hot bath, combined with the use of aromatic oils, will help you to feel calm and relaxed and encourage you to slow down.

Sea Mineral Bath

Taking a sea mineral bath is like soaking in a warm tropical ocean. Soak in a bath of sea minerals to nourish, cleanse, and rejuvenate the cells of your skin.

Dissolve three to four pounds of sea salt (you can buy it in bulk at most health food stores) in a tub of hot water. Relax and soak for twenty minutes. Just as saltwater cleanses your skin, salt air opens, refreshes, and cleanses the breathing passages. As you soak in your bath, try practicing one of the simple breathing techniques described in Day Six.

Adding essential oils to your bath offers a wide range of possibilities for relaxation, rejuvenation, and healing. Essential oils are readily absorbed by the skin, and inhaling their fragrance in steam also affects both the mind and the body.

Tranquility Bath

Draw a hot bath and add

7 drops of lavender essential oil
10 drops of chamomile essential oil
5 drops of marjoram essential oil

Lavender and chamomile soothe tension, and marjoram relieves tight muscles.

BODY SCRUBS

You may want to use a body scrub to exfoliate your skin and bring circulation to the surface of the skin. While you can purchase a variety of body scrubs on the market, it can be interesting and much more cost-effective to make them yourself. It is a good idea to make a cup at a time to see if you like the scent and texture. The formula is simple: Combine two parts salt (e.g., sea salt, kosher salt, or Epsom salt) with one part beauty oil (e.g., almond, apricot, or grape seed oil) along with several drops of your favorite essential oil (see above for a listing of essential oils and their effects).

DRY BRUSHING

One of the most effective aids to detoxification is dry brushing, which involves brushing the skin with a natural bristle brush when your skin is dry. Dry brushing takes advantage of the cleansing function of the skin by lifting off the surface cells to open the pores and let your skin breathe. It also brings heat and circulation to the surface of the skin. Most important, dry brushing stimulates the lymphatic system, which moves waste through the body to the eliminative organs and lymphatic drainage sites. Using a natural bristle skin brush every day is one of the best ways to aid in the release of toxins and assist your body in cleansing.

Dry brushing must be done when your body is dry, not while you are in the bath or the shower. It is best to do your dry brushing in the morning, prior to exercising or taking a bath or shower, but you also can do it in the evening before you go to sleep. Starting with the soles of your feet, gently brush your body using long, light, upward strokes. Brush from the feet to the ankles to the calves, concentrating on the area behind the knees. Then brush from the knees to the thighs and torso, finally making long strokes from the wrists to the shoulders and underarms. This should take no more that three to five minutes.

You can find natural bristle skin brushes at most health food stores. Some are far too rough, and I prefer the body brush by Bass.

MASSAGE

As mentioned earlier, massage can be a wonderful aid in the cleansing process because it enhances circulation, releases tension and lactic acid stored in the muscles, stimulates the lymphatic system, and assists in the removal of toxins. If you can fit in a few deep tissue massage sessions during this cleanse, it will be very helpful.

In addition, other healing modalities, alternative therapies, and energy work such as acupuncture, chiropractic work, craniosacral therapy, and Reiki also may enhance your experience and optimize the effects of the cleanse.

RECIPES FOR DAY FOURTEEN

Cucumber-Celery Juice

3-4 stalks celery
½ cucumber
Juice all ingredients in a juicer, and drink immediately.

Pyncnogenol Passion Smoothie

1 cascade red or black grapes, preferably with seeds
1 cup cherries, pitted and frozen
½ cup Manuka or Thompson raisins, soaked one hour in ½ cup water—reserve the soak water
½ avocado
2 cups fresh apple juice
2 tablespoons flax seed oil—optional
Pluck grapes from stem and freeze, or use at room temperature. Blend all ingredients together in a blender until smooth, about two minutes. Make sure that the seeds are completely ground. Spoon into sorbet glasses.

Creamy Carrot-Ginger Soup

(Makes 2 servings)

1½ cups fresh carrot juice

½ small avocado

⅓ cup coconut meat from a fresh, young coconut

1 tablespoon lime juice

2 teaspoons minced ginger

Pinch of cayenne pepper

Pinch of sea salt

A few sprigs of cilantro for garnish

Blend all ingredients in a blender until smooth. Garnish with cilantro leaves.

Avocado and Apple Salad with Wakame

(Makes 2 servings)

2 teaspoons extra-virgin olive oil

½ teaspoon lemon juice

Sea salt and pepper to taste

½ avocado, thinly sliced

½ apple, peeled, cored, and julienned

2 teaspoons wakame, soaked for twenty to thirty minutes, drained, and julienned

Whisk together the olive oil and lemon juice. Season with salt and pepper. Add the avocado, apple, and wakame. Toss gently.

Garden Herb Roll-ups

(Makes 2 servings)

For the Wraps:

3 large collard leaves

2 Roma tomatoes, thinly sliced

For the Pumpkin Seed Pâté:

1 clove garlic

¼ cup Brazil nuts

¼ cup lemon juice

1½ cups pumpkin seeds, soaked for four to six hours, drained, and rinsed

¼ cup olive oil

½ teaspoon salt

2 tablespoons parsley

2 tablespoons basil

3 tablespoons dill

Chop the garlic in a food processor. Add the Brazil nuts and process until they are finely chopped. With the blade running, add the lemon juice until the mixture is creamy. Add the pumpkin seeds, the olive oil, and the sea salt and continue to puree this mixture. Add the parsley, basil, and dill and pulse to finely chop the herbs.

For the Marinated Veggies:

1 cup baby spinach

¾ cup shredded carrots

2 tablespoons onion, very thinly sliced

1 tablespoon extra-virgin olive oil

1 teaspoon lemon juice

Pinch of sea salt

Freshly ground black pepper to taste

Toss all ingredients in a large bowl, and mix well to combine all the flavors.

For the Assembly:

Lay a collard green on your cutting board with the darker side on the board. Chop off the stem, and trim off any very thick portions of the remaining center stem. Place 6 tablespoons of the pâté on the collard leaf and spread it out a bit, but leave plenty of room for wrapping up the leaf. Top with a few slices of tomato. Cover with ½ cup of the marinated veggies. Roll up like a burrito, folding up the top and bottom first and then rolling in the sides.

DAY
FIFTEEN

When we accept what is in this very moment, without pushing
or pulling, when there is no running after or running away, we
find in our practice a level of deep acceptance and peace.
—*Michael Stone*

Please remember to think of this last phase of the cleanse as a week of *indulgence:* Feast
on as much luscious fruit and vibrant vegetables as possible, explore some raw-food
creations, and observe how your body feels with all this living energy passing through.
It is a good time to turn inward, in a joyful way, to fully experience the effects of these
changes you are taking on.

I encourage you to make the next week a kind of internal pilgrimage: Travel the
landscape of your mind and body to discover the truth that lies at your innermost being. The meditation practices and exercises for the next few days will focus on this idea of
tuning into our thoughts, feelings, and physical sensations to generate mindfulness and
to touch the inherent joy that such mindfulness brings.

Exercise for Day Fifteen

OPEN AWARENESS

Sit comfortably in a quiet place. Bring awareness to your breath. Observe your thoughts and feelings. Notice with interest and ease all that
presents itself to you. As you sit, sense your ability to rest calmly and
solidly through the seasons of life change. Remain sitting this way for
some time, aware of your capacity to be open, alive, and present to all
that arises.

Yoga Pose for Day Fifteen
BOW POSE (*DANURASANA*)

Benefits: Stretches and strengthens the back muscles, lengthens the abdominal and chest muscles, stretches the quadriceps, and strengthens the legs.

Do not do this pose if you are pregnant because it places too much pressure on
the abdomen. Lie on your belly with your forehead resting on the floor. Bend
your knees, and reach back to hold your ankles in your hands. Press your upper thighs and lower abdomen down into the floor. Flex your feet, and lift your
knees up off the floor. Rest on your abdomen, and attempt to straighten the
legs while holding the ankles. Take three to five long, deep breaths. Release
your ankles and lie on the front of your body with one cheek resting on the
floor. It is helpful to repeat this pose two or three consecutive times.

THE NUTRITIONAL BENEFITS OF RAW VEGETABLES

As you know, raw food is full of healthy nutrients, vitamins, minerals, and enzymes.
The raw foods we eat during this final phase of our cleanse should be easy to digest, so
fresh fruit juices and vegetable juices and blended fruit and green smoothies can play
an important role. If at all possible, the raw foods you eat should be organic so as to be
completely free from any pesticides or fertilizer residue.

Since in these last days of our cleanse vegetables are a predominant component of
our diet, I thought I would share this listing of some vegetables and their nutritional
properties.

Leafy Greens

Bok choy has anti-inflammatory, anticancer, and antioxidant properties and is high in
calcium.

Cabbage provides fiber to cleanse the digestive tract and alleviate constipation. Its sulfur
and chlorine content cleanses the mucous membrane of the stomach and intestinal tract,
and its high levels of vitamin C strengthen the immune system. Cabbage is both antibacterial and antiviral, which makes it effective in killing germs, parasites, and viruses.
Cabbage is also high in vitamin K, iodine, iron, manganese, and fiber.

Celery has a high percentage of organic sodium, which is vital to many bodily functions and guards against dehydration. Celery is also high in magnesium and iron, which makes it valuable for blood cells. Celery also provides vitamin C and helps to prevent cancer and to lower cholesterol and blood pressure. It is highly alkaline and acts as a diuretic and a blood cleanser.

Chard is high in beta-carotene, vitamin K, vitamin C, vitamin E, copper, magnesium, iron, manganese, phosphorus, potassium, selenium, sodium, and zinc.

Collards have anti-inflammatory, anticancer, antioxidant, and alkaline qualities. They are high in sulfur, folate, vitamin C, vitamin K, vitamins B_1, B_2, B_3, B_5, and B_6, vitamin E, copper, magnesium, potassium, iron, manganese, phosphorus, potassium, calcium, selenium, sodium, zinc, and fiber.

Dandelion is a blood cleanser, detoxifier, and digestive aid. It contains high levels of beta-carotene, vitamin C, vitamins B_1, B_2, and B_6, vitamin K, vitamin E, folate, copper, magnesium, potassium, iron, manganese, phosphorus, potassium, calcium, sodium, zinc, fiber, and omega-6.

Kale is an exceptional source of calcium, iron, sulfur, chlorophyll, and vitamin A, and its beta-carotene content far outweighs that of spinach. Kale has a cleansing, antiviral, and anticancer effect. It is a rich source of vitamin C, vitamins B_1, B_2, B_3, B_5, and B_6, beta-carotene, vitamin K, lutein, copper, magnesium, iron, manganese, phosphorus, potassium, selenium, sodium, zinc, and sulfur.

Lettuce (romaine, red leaf, and butter lettuce) is rich in vitamin E, folate, vitamin C, vitamins B_1 and B_2, vitamin K, copper, magnesium, potassium, iron, manganese, phosphorus, and calcium.

Spinach is nutrient-dense and enriches the blood owing to its high iron and chlorophyll content. It also stops bleeding and is used as a specific remedy for nosebleeds and herpes. Spinach is also a potent laxative and diuretic and cleanses the blood of toxins. It provides high doses of beta-carotene, folate, vitamin K, vitamins B_1, B_2, and B_6, vitamin C, vitamin E, calcium, copper, iron, magnesium, manganese, potassium, sodium, zinc, and omega-3.

Root Vegetables

Beets cleanse the kidneys and the digestive system. They are high in copper, magnesium, iron, manganese, and potassium.

Carrots are believed to enhance blood flow to the eyes and thereby improve eyesight and night vision. They are one of the richest sources of beta-carotene and may protect against cancer, dissolve accumulations such as stones and tumors, and help with ear infections, earaches, and deafness. They are alkalizing, cleansing, and nourishing and are rich in beta-carotene, vitamins, minerals, enzymes, and fiber.

Fennel supports the digestive system and contains folate, vitamin B_5, vitamin C, calcium, potassium, magnesium, manganese, phosphorus, iron, and copper.

Jicama provides vitamin C, copper, and iron.

Onions are antiseptic, anticoagulant, detoxifying, and diuretic. They act as an expectorant, a stimulant, and an overall tonic. Onions are effective in preventing cancer, and they provide folate, vitamins B_1 and B_6, vitamin C, sulfur, manganese, copper, and zinc.

Parsnips are a detoxifier, a cleanser, and a diuretic. They contain high levels of fiber, folate, vitamins B_1 and B_5, vitamin C, vitamin E, manganese, and copper.

Radishes are antibacterial, antifungal, diuretic, and stimulating. They offer folate, vitamin C, copper, iron, and zinc.

Turnips are anticancer, antioxidant, antibiotic, and antiviral. They provide sulfur, B vitamins, vitamin C, copper, manganese, and sodium.

Starchy Vegetables

Corn is rich in folate, vitamin C, vitamins B_1, B_2, B_3, B_5, and B_6, copper, magnesium, iron, manganese, phosphorus, potassium, selenium, sodium, zinc, and fiber. Please take care to avoid genetically modified (GMO) corn.

Peas are a blood sugar regulator containing lectins, folate, beta-carotene, vitamins B_1, B_2, B_3, and B_6, vitamin C, vitamin K, copper, manganese, phosphorus, iron, zinc, and fiber.

Pumpkin reduces inflammation and is thought to lower lung and prostate cancer risk. It acts as a diuretic and a laxative and provides beta-carotene, vitamin B_2, vitamin C, vitamin E, copper, iron, and potassium.

Squash (winter squash, acorn, Hubbard) is beneficial for eyesight and heart function. It is alkalizing and contains beta-carotene, vitamins B_1, B_5, and B_6, vitamin C, copper, iron, magnesium, manganese, phosphorus, and potassium.

Sweet potato is a detoxifier that provides digestive support and is good for the eyes. It has anticancer and antioxidant properties and provides beta-carotene, vitamins B_1, B_5, and B_6, copper, iron, magnesium, manganese, phosphorus, and potassium.

Zucchini is also alkalizing and offers beta-carotene, vitamins B_1, B_3, B_5, and B_6, vitamin C, copper, iron, magnesium, manganese, phosphorus, potassium, and zinc.

Miscellaneous Vegetables

Asparagus is a diuretic and a laxative, and it cleanses the kidneys, is believed to promote healthy bacteria in the gut, improves heart health, and provides vitamin C, beta-carotene, folic acid, vitamins B_1, B_2, and B_3, and fiber.

Broccoli lowers the risk of prostate, bladder, colon, pancreatic, gastric, and breast cancers and provides vitamin C, folate, vitamins B_1, B_2, B_3, B_5, and B_6, vitamin K, copper, magnesium, iron, manganese, potassium, calcium, selenium, sodium, zinc, sulfur, and fiber.

Cauliflower is a blood purifier that contains sulfur, fiber, cancer-preventing antioxidants, vitamin C, folate, vitamin K, copper, magnesium, potassium, iron, manganese, calcium, selenium, sodium, and zinc.

Okra is soothing to the digestive tract and provides copper, magnesium, iron, manganese, phosphorus, potassium, calcium, and zinc.

Peppers (sweet red peppers as well as hot peppers) are antibacterial, antiseptic, and stimulating. They provide circulatory support, discourage certain parasites, and contain capsaicin, beta-carotene, vitamin C, vitamin B$_6$, copper, iron, manganese, magnesium, and omega-6.

Radicchio is rich in folate, vitamin C, vitamin E, copper, iron, and zinc.

RECIPES FOR DAY FIFTEEN

Apple-Strawberry Juice

2 apples

4–6 strawberries

Juice all ingredients in a juicer, and drink immediately.

Strawberry-Banana-Romaine Smoothie

1 cup strawberries

2 bananas

½ bunch romaine

2 cups water

Blend all ingredients together in a blender until smooth.

Broccoli Soup

(Makes 3 servings)

2 tablespoons raw sunflower seeds, soaked for at least thirty minutes and rinsed

3 shitake mushrooms, fresh or dried

2 teaspoons Nama Shoyu soy sauce

½ head celery

1 inch fresh ginger

1 cucumber

1 lemon, peel removed

1½ cups broccoli tops

1 tomato

1 garlic clove, peeled

2 tablespoons extra-virgin olive oil

2 tablespoons raw sesame tahini

¼ cup red onion, diced

Pinch of cayenne pepper to taste

½ cup water

1 sprig fresh cilantro

If using dried shitake mushrooms, combine the 2 tea-spoons Nama Shoyu soy sauce with ¼ cup of water and soak for at least one hour. If using fresh mushrooms, mari-nate them in the 2 teaspoons of soy sauce for one hour. Remove the mushrooms from the marinade and set aside. Juice celery, ginger, cucumber, and lemon in a juicer. Add the juice to the remaining ingredients, including the soy sauce marinade. Blend all ingredients in a blender until smooth. Garnish with the marinated mushrooms and a few cilantro leaves.

· ·

Carrot-Raisin Salad

4 large carrots, grated

½ cup raisins

Juice of ½ lemon

Soak the raisins in water for at least ½ hour. Combine grated carrots with the soaked raisins and lemon juice, and mix together before serving.

· ·

Mushroom and Cherry Tomato Fettucini

(Makes 2 servings)

1–2 goldbar squashes, ends trimmed (or substitute an-other summer squash or zucchini)

Sea salt to taste

1 cup cherry tomatoes, sliced in half

1–2 tablespoons extra-virgin olive oil

Freshly ground black pepper

1 cup mushrooms (field mushrooms with a dense texture work best)

1 teaspoon balsamic vinegar

1 teaspoon Nama Shoyu soy sauce

1–2 whole stalks fresh rosemary

Small handful fresh oregano or 1 teaspoon dried oregano

1 shallot, minced

Using a vegetable peeler or mandoline, slice the squash

into wide, thin, fettucine noodle–like ribbons. Discard the seeds at the center. Toss the sliced squash in a colander with ½ teaspoon sea salt. Allow to sit for at least thirty minutes to allow some of the liquid to drain out.

Toss the cherry tomatoes with 1 tablespoon of the olive oil, and season with salt and pepper. Toss well and allow to marinate for several hours.

Toss the mushrooms with 1 tablespoon of the olive oil, the balsamic vinegar, and the Nama Shoyu soy sauce. Season with salt and pepper. Add rosemary, oregano, and shallot. Toss well and allow to marinate for several hours.

Toss the squash noodles with the mushroom mixture and the cherry tomatoes. Season with salt and pepper and garnish with fresh herbs.

DAY
SIXTEEN

Following a spiritual path can be a little like falling in love.
When you are in love, the beloved's presence colors every
experience.

—Lama Miller

I hope that you are inspired to take these next steps toward greater physical and spiritual health. I encourage you to continue to kindle enthusiasm for the journey. If you can bring the excitement of new love to your everyday walk with life, then even your mundane daily activities can be imbued with freshness and beauty, and life becomes an adventure. Today, see if you can allow your routine tasks to be colored by wonder and joy, as if you are doing them for the very first time.

Exercise for Day Sixteen

AWAKENING IN OUR EVERYDAY ACTIONS

Choose a simple, repetitive activity—washing the dishes, folding the laundry, walking the dog, brushing your teeth. While doing this activity, seek to become completely involved. Allow yourself to be totally absorbed, to the point of feeling as though you are one with the activity. Notice how rich your experience becomes if you embrace it with the wide-eyed wonder of a child or with the infectious enthusiasm of new love.

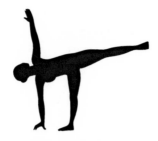

Yoga Pose for Day Sixteen

HALF-MOON POSE
(*ARDHA CHANDRASANA*)

Benefits: Improves balance, stretches the hamstrings, opens the hip joints, strengthens the thighs, and allows the chest to expand.

Avoid this pose if you are feeling shaky or unstable. You may chose to practice with your back against a wall for support if you feel unsteady. Stand with your feet about one leg's length apart. Come into Triangle Pose with the right foot in front (see Day Thirteen). Step the left foot a few inches toward the right foot. Bring your right fingertips to the floor eight to ten inches in front of your right pinkie toe. Straighten your right leg as you lift your left leg up to hip height, parallel to the floor. Work to stack your hips and shoulders. Hold the pose for several full, relaxed breaths. Repeat on the other side.

SOAKING AND SPROUTING NUTS AND SEEDS

Since you will not be eating animal products or cooked food during this final week of the cleanse, nuts, seeds, and sprouts, although best consumed in moderation, may be a helpful component of your all-raw diet.

Raw nuts and seeds, whole or in their sprouted form, are good sources protein and also provide healthy fat and fiber. It is beneficial to soak nuts and seeds mainly because they contain enzyme inhibitors that protect the nut or seed until it has what it needs for growing. Nature works so miraculously. When it rains, the nuts or seeds get enough moisture to germinate and produce a plant. The inhibitors are released, and the plant then continues to grow with the sunlight.

By soaking nuts and seeds, you increase the life and vitality contained within them while also releasing the toxic enzyme inhibitors. Soaking also increases the availability of vitamins and breaks down the gluten so that digestion is much easier. Best of all, sprouting allows you to have a garden in your own kitchen and enables you to grow your own protein-rich living food.

It is easiest to sprout seeds or nuts in glass gallon- or half-gallon-sized Ball jars or similar-style Mason jars. You can use a flexible mesh screen from a hardware store with a ring lid to secure the mesh tightly or purchase plastic sprouting lids that have the mesh tops built in. You may soak, sprout, rinse, and drain your nuts and seeds in these jars. The following table lists the amounts and sprouting times for various seeds, nuts, and legumes.

Soaking and Sprouting Times

Nut/Seed	Dry Amount	Soak Time	Sprout Time	Sprout Length	Yield
Alfalfa seed	3 tbsp	12 hours	3–5 days	1–2 inches	4 cups
Almonds	3 cups	8–12 hours	1–3 days	⅛ inch	4 cups
Amaranth	1 cup	3–5 hours	2–3 days	¼ inch	3 cups
Barley, hulless	1 cup	6 hours	12–24 hours	¼ inch	2 cups
Broccoli seed	2 tbsp	8 hours	3–4 days	1–2 inches	2 cups
Buckwheat, hulled	1 cup	6 hours	1–2 days	⅛–½ inch	2 cups
Cabbage seed	1 tbsp	4–6 hours	4–5 days	1–2 inches	1½ cups
Cashews	3 cups	2–3 hours	—	N/A	4 cups
Clover	3 tbsp	5 hours	4–6 days	1–2 inches	4 cups
Fenugreek	4 tbsp	6 hours	2–5 days	1–2 inches	3 cups
Flax seeds	1 cup	6 hours	N/A	—	2 cups
Garbanzo beans (chick peas)	1 cup	12–48 hours	2–4 days	½–1 inch	4 cups
Kale seed	4 tbsp	4–6 hours	4–6 days	¾–1 inch	3–4 cups
Lentils	3/4 cup	8 hours	2–3 days	½–1 inch	4 cups
Millet	1 cup	5 hours	12 hours	¹⁄₁₆ inch	3 cups
Mung beans	1/3 cup	8 hours	4–5 days	¼–3 inches	4 cups
Mustard seed	3 tbsp	5 hours	3–5 days	½–1½ inches	3 cups
Oats, hulled	1 cup	8 hours	1–2 days	⅛ inch	1 cup
Onion seed	1 tbsp	4-6 hours	4–5 days	1–2 inches	1½–2 cups
Peas	1 cup	8 hours	2–3 days	½–1 inch	3 cups
Pinto beans	1 cup	12 hours	3–4 days	½–1 inch	3–4 cups
Pumpkin	1 cup	6 hours	1–2 days	⅛ inch	2 cups
Quinoa	1 cup	3–4 hours	2–3 days	½ inch	3 cups
Radish	3 tbsp	6 hours	3–5 days	¾–2 inches	4 cups
Rye	1 cup	6–8 hours	2–3 days	½–¾ inch	3 cups

Sesame seed, hulled	1 cup	8 hours	—	N/A	1½ cups
Sesame seed, unhulled	1 cup	4–6 hours	1–2 days	⅛ inch	1 cup
Spelt	1 cup	6 hours	1–2 days	¼ inch	3 cups
Sunflower, hulled	1 cup	6–8 hours	1 day	¼–½ inch	2 cups
Teff	1 cup	3–4 hours	1–2 days	⅛ inch	3 cups
Walnuts	3 cups	4 hours	N/A	—	4 cups
Wheat	1 cup	8–12 hours	2–3 days	¼–¾ inch	3 cups
Wild rice	1 cup	12 hours	2–3 days	Rice spits	3 cups

General Procedure for Sprouting

After placing the water and the nuts/seeds/legumes in the jar, let them soak for the pre-scribed time. Then drain the water well by placing the jar upside down in the sink for ten minutes. Put the jar in a dark place, face down, at an angle, covered with a towel for the appropriate length of time. Positioning the jar in a dish rack or a high-rimmed bowl works well because it allows the excess water to drain out. Rinse two to three times a day by filling the jar with water, shaking vigorously, and draining it well. Be sure to drain the jar well. Seeds that sit in water can spoil the whole jar. Let the sprouts grow for the suggested number of days. On the last day of sprouting time, put the jar in the sun (indirect sunlight is best) not necessarily outdoors—on a kitchen counter is fine—until the sprouts turn green and are ready to eat. Continue to rinse the growing sprouts two to three times daily, draining the jar completely after each rinse.

After the final rinse, let the sprouts dry completely. They should be dry to the touch. If the sprouts are even slightly moist, they will die quickly in the refrigerator. The sprouts then can be stored in the refrigerator for up to six weeks.

You can buy the sprouting seeds and other equipment at most health food stores or purchase them online. As you can see in the table, the soaking times vary with the nut or seed. Generally, the more dense the seed or nut, the longer is the soaking time. Ideally, soaking should be done at room temperature.

RECIPES FOR DAY SIXTEEN

. . . .

Citrus Cleansing Juice

¼ lemon with peel

½ grapefruit, peeled

2 oranges, peeled

Juice all ingredients in a juicer, and drink immediately.

. . . .

Dark Green Smoothie

(Makes 1 quart)

½ bunch dandelion greens

2 Roma tomatoes

1½ cups water

Blend all ingredients together in a blender until smooth.

. . . .

Pepper Soup

(Makes 2 servings)

1 yellow bell pepper, cored and chopped

1 red bell pepper, cored and chopped

1 green bell pepper, cored and chopped

1 large tomato, diced

½ cup parsley or cliantro (or a blend of both), chopped

½ cup basil leaves, loosely packed

¼ cup onion, chopped

½ apple, cored and chopped

½ cup raw sesame seeds, freshly ground in a coffee grinder or food processor

2 tablespoons unpasteurized miso

3 tablespoons raw apple cider vinegar

¼ cup Bragg's liquid aminos or Nama Shoyu soy sauce

½ habanero pepper

½ teaspoon salt

Freshly ground black pepper to taste

2 cups water

Blend all ingredients in a blender until smooth.

* *

"Pizza" Salad

(Makes 2 servings)

6–8 unsulfured sun-dried tomatoes, soaked in lukewarm water until soft, chopped

¼–½ pound fresh baby greens

¼ cup fresh basil, chopped

1 tablespoon fresh oregano, chopped

1 tablespoon lemon juice

1 clove garlic, minced—optional

1 teaspoon raw honey or raw agave nectar—optional

Sea salt and freshly ground black pepper to taste

Combine all the ingredients, and toss well.

* *

Zucchini and Tomato Lasagne

(Makes 3 servings)

For the Pine Nut "Ricotta":

1 cup raw pine (pignoli) nuts, soaked for at least one hour

1 tablespoon lemon juice

1 tablespoon nutritional yeast

½ teaspoon sea salt

1–2 tablespoons water

Place pine nuts, nutritional yeast, lemon juice, and salt in a food processor, and pulse until combined. Add water gradually, and process until the mixture resembles ricotta cheese.

For the Tomato Sauce:

1 cup sun-dried tomatoes, soaked for at least two hours

½ small to medium tomato, diced

2 tablespoons onion, chopped fine

1 tablespoon lemon juice

2 tablespoons extra-virgin olive oil

2 teaspoons raw agave nectar

1 teaspoon sea salt

Drain soaked sun-dried tomatoes, and add to blender, along with remaining ingredients. Blend all ingredients until smooth.

For the Pesto:

1 cup basil leaves, packed

¼ cup raw pistachios

3 tablespoons extra-virgin olive oil

½ teaspoon sea salt

Freshly ground black pepper to taste

Blend in food processor until combined but still chunky.

For the Assembly:

1–2 medium zucchini

1 tablespoon extra-virgin olive oil

2 teaspoons fresh oregano, finely chopped

2 teaspoons fresh thyme

Pinch of sea salt

Pinch of freshly ground black pepper

2 medium tomatoes, cut in half and then sliced

Whole basil leaves for garnish

Cut the zucchini into three-inch lengths. Cut lengthwise into very thin slices using a mandoline or a vegetable peeler. Toss the zucchini slices with the olive oil, oregano, thyme, and salt and pepper.

Line the bottom of a nine- by thirteen-inch backing dish with a layer of zucchini slices, overlapping the slices slightly. Spread about a third of the tomato sauce over the slices, and top with small dollops of the pine nut "ricotta" mixture and the pesto, using about a third of each. Layer on a third of the tomato slices. Add another layer of the zucchini slices, and repeat twice more. You may serve immediately or cover with plastic wrap and allow to sit at room temperature for several hours. Garnish with basil leaves.

DAY SEVENTEEN

> When the mind turns to others, it is engaging in something
> that is extraordinary. What it is about to do is amazing. It
> is going to step outside, away from itself, and be less self-
> concerned.
>
> —*Sakyong Mipham Rinpoche*

As you draw near the end of the cleanse, it is fitting to remind yourself that your practice of yoga, your exploration of meditation, and your foray into this cleanse are borne of a desire to be of benefit to yourself and others. Today, I suggest that you draw special attention to the *others* in that aspiration by focusing on thoughts, feelings, and actions that are other-centered.

We begin to cultivate a compassionate heart—a heart without limits—by first developing self-understanding and self-acceptance. Then we continue the process by shifting our focus away from ourselves, which is where it usually points, and directing it toward others. And not just others in theory, but others as the people with whom we actually have direct contact in our lives.

Shifting your focus from your own concerns to the concerns of others simply requires that you ask yourself:

What if I were in his or her place?
What if his or her happiness were as important as my own?

The small discomforts that this final phase of the cleanse might bring—your extra efforts to practice yoga and meditation, to use your breath to grow awareness, to get outdoors and appreciate beauty, to feel gratitude for life's many gifts—all of these can be humble offerings that spring from the positive desire to be of help to yourself and especially to others.

Exercise for Day Seventeen

OTHER-CENTERED

Today, notice when you feel irritated or annoyed with someone, even just mildly so. When you encounter this situation, ask yourself

How does this person with whom I am irritated experience this moment?
How does it really feel to be this person right now?
What is he or she thinking or feeling?

Put your own feelings aside temporarily, and take the other person's place. Shift your perspective and see where that goes.

Yoga Pose for Day Seventeen

FISH POSE (*MATSYASANA*)

Benefits: Opens the front of the neck and the abdomen,
stretches the muscles of the throat, strengthens the upper
back and the back of the neck, and improves posture.

Do not practice this pose if you have migraine headaches or neck or low-back injuries. Lie on your back with your knees bent, feet on the floor. Inhale, lift your pelvis slightly off the floor, and slide your hands, palms down, below your buttocks. Then rest your buttocks on the backs of your hands. Do not lift your buttocks up off of your hands as you perform this pose. Please note that the above illustration shows the hips and legs lifted up off the floor but that is an advanced version of the pose which places excessive pressure on the neck. Instead, keep your buttocks resting on your hands. Place your forearms and elbows close to the sides of your torso. Press into your elbows. Lift your chest and drop your head back so that the crown of your head rests on the floor. Keep your knees bent, or straighten your legs out onto the floor. Take five to eight deep, smooth breaths.

By way of review, on a raw-food diet you want to

Maximize your intake of

—**fresh fruits and vegetables.** This means pretty much any fresh fruits or vegetables, and the fresher the better. Once the food is picked, its vitality immediately begins to decrease. Refrigeration reduces the vitality even further. If you can pick the produce yourself, that is ideal. The next-best choice is to buy directly from a farmer or farmers' market. The next-best choice is to purchase your raw produce from a health food store. The least favorable option is to buy from a larger grocery chain store.

—**fresh sprouts.** You may purchase sprouted seeds at a health food store or purchase the seeds and sprout them yourself and eat these life-force-rich foods while they are still living and growing. Day Sixteen contains more information about sprouting.

Moderate your intake of

—**nuts and seeds.** Many nuts are raw and go through no heat processing. Purchase nuts in the shell whenever possible because once nuts are out of the shell, they start to oxidize and can become rancid quite easily. Some nuts are heated in the process of extracting the nut from the shell.

A note about cashews: Unfortunately, most cashew nuts labeled "raw" are not truly raw. They have been heat processed—usually steamed and boiled in oil—in order to remove the nut from the toxic shell. Many people avoid cashew nuts because of their high fat content, although they are lower in total fat than almonds, peanuts, pecans, and walnuts. That said, cashews provide essential fatty acids, B vitamins, fiber, protein, carbohydrates, potassium, iron, and zinc. Like other nuts, cashews have a small percentage of saturated fat, but eaten in small quantities, cashews are a nutritious food.

—**young coconuts.** Young coconuts are an excellent source of electrolytes, fat, and calcium.

—**dried fruits.** Technically, only sun-dried foods would be considered raw because they are dried by the sun. Most dried fruits that you find in the health food store (including sun-dried tomatoes) are heated to a temperature well over 200°F.

—**dates.** If you purchase good organic dates, they are generally sun-dried. Many "conventional" dates are dried and then steamed to make them plump and moist, so they would not qualify as a raw food.

—**seaweed.** Many small "family" businesses sun-dry their seaweed, such as nori, dulse, laver, sea lettuce, wakame, and kombu. Seaweeds produced and packaged by larger companies may or may not be sun-dried. Sometimes they are roasted, and that is not always mentioned on the packaging.

—**dried vegetables, herbs, and spices.** It is uncertain whether these have been heat treated in the drying process. Whenever possible, it is best to use fresh herbs and spices or dry the spices yourself.

—**olives.** Most olives are preserved with salt and packed in a vinegar or lactic acid brine, neither of which is recommended on a cleansing diet. Canned olives usually are cooked in the canning process. The best raw olives are sun-dried raw olives, which are difficult to find but worth the effort if you enjoy the taste of olives.

—**green powders.** A good green food powder can be somewhat helpful as long as it is not heat-processed and instead is dried at a low temperature and does not include toxic additives. However, green powders should be seen as a supplement and not as a substitute for fresh green juices or smoothies.

—**raw honey.** While it is best to minimize your use of concentrated sweeteners, raw honey is a good choice for its healing properties, although it is not accepted by strict vegans.

—**frozen fruits.** Most frozen fruits are not blanched before freezing, so they are considered "raw." However, it is ideal to eat fresh fruit or freeze fruits yourself.

Minimize your intake of the following items (even though these items are often included in a raw-food diet, and while they are not harmful in moderation, it is healthier to minimize their use over the longer term):

—**table salt and sea salt.** While table salt is much worse than Celtic sea salt, we get enough sodium from fruits, vegetables, and seaweed, so it is best to use even sea salt in moderation.

—**Nama Shoyu soy sauce, tamari, and Bragg's liquid aminos.** These are fine to use sparingly, but bear in mind that they are highly processed, fermented foods that are acid-forming and toxic to the body if consumed in excess. A dash of seaweed powder (i.e., kelp, dulse, or nori) is a much healthier seasoning alternative.

—**maple syrup.** All maple syrup is cooked, so it is never raw. Since dates taste a lot like maple syrup, they are an excellent substitute. Simply blend pitted dates with some water to create a syrup.

—**bottled oils.** Once oil is extracted from its original source, it generally turns rancid very quickly. Even cold-pressed organic oils are extremely concentrated and difficult for our bodies to break down. As a rule, it is better to eat the food instead—that is, olives instead of olive oil, coconuts instead of coconut oil, ground flax seeds instead of flax oil.

—**frozen vegetables.** Most frozen vegetables are blanched before they are quick frozen, so they do not qualify as raw food.

RECIPES FOR DAY SEVENTEEN

Alkalizing Juice

¼ head cabbage, red or green
3 stalks celery
Juice all ingredients in a juicer, and drink immediately.

Dark Green Smoothie

(Makes 1 quart)
½ bunch dandelion greens
2 Roma tomatoes
1½ cups water
Blend all ingredients together in a blender until smooth.

Papaya-Mint Bisque

(Makes 2 servings)

2 tablespoons fresh mint leaves, torn

1 large or 2 small Hawaiian papayas, chilled and seeded

¼–⅓ cup water

1 lime, juiced

1 tablespoon fresh pineapple or fresh orange juice

Puree all ingredients in a food processor until smooth. Garnish with mint leaves and halved red grapes.

Thai Cucumber Salad

1 cucumber, chopped

2 Roma tomatoes, diced

½ avocado, chopped

½ cup sun-dried tomatoes, soaked four hours, drained, and diced

2 mint leaves, minced

2 basil leaves, minced

½ teaspoon fresh finely diced ginger

Juice of 1 lime

2 tablespoons hemp seeds

Toss all ingredients together in a bowl.

Green Curry Coconut Noodles

(Makes 2 to 4 servings)

For the Vegetables:

2 tablespoons extra-virgin olive oil

2 tablespoons white miso

2 teaspoons raw apple cider vinegar

1 tablespoon chopped ginger

1 teaspoon sesame oil

1 green onion, thinly sliced

½ cup yellow squash, thinly sliced

½ cup zucchini, thinly sliced

½ cup mushrooms, diced small

½ carrot, cut into matchsticks

½ cup sliced snap peas, cut on a diagonal into diamond shapes

½ small stalk celery, cut in half lengthwise and then sliced thin

In a blender, puree the miso, vinegar, ginger, sesame oil, and half the green onion until smooth. Add the second half of the thinly sliced green onion, and toss the sauce with the vegetables. Allow to marinate for at least three hours.

For the Curry:

2 tablespoons grated lemongrass

½ cup coconut meat

2 tablespoons raw cashews, soaked for at least one hour

1 tablespoon lime juice

2 tablespoons chopped jalepeno pepper

2 green onions

1 tablespoon chopped ginger

2 tablespoons basil, loosly packed

1 teaspoons curry powder

1 teaspoon sea salt

¼ cup coconut water

Place all ingredients except coconut water in a blender, and blend until smooth. Add coconut water a bit at a time until the mixture is the consistency of a thick sauce.

For the Assembly:

¼ cup chopped almonds

½ teaspoon sesame oil

¼ teaspoon sea salt

1 cup coconut "noodles" (from four coconuts)

1 small handful cilantro, chopped

2 tablespoons mint, chopped or torn

2 tablespoons basil, chopped or torn

1 tablespoon sesame seeds, preferably black

Toss almonds with sesame oil and sea salt.

Add coconut "noodles" to vegetables, add herbs, and toss to combine. Sprinkle with chopped almonds and sesame seeds. Serve with curry sauce.

DAY
EIGHTEEN

Every act counts. Every thought and emotion counts, too. This
is all the path we have.

—*Pema Chodron*

We often move through our days in a reactive way, going through the motions in a dis-connected state of mind. We forget that we can choose to be conscious and deliberate about what we are thinking and doing in each present moment. Consider the statement: "If you want to know where you have been in the past, look at your mind now. If you want to look at where you are going in the future, look at your actions now."

There is power in the present moment. Now is in fact the only time we have. How we relate to it creates our future. As you enter these final days of the cleanse, it is helpful to remember how potent your current, real-time thoughts and actions are. They propel you on your way. Today, spend some time looking at your actions. Ask yourself what they tell you.

Exercise for Day Eighteen

OBSERVE YOUR ACTIONS

If you want to know where you have been in the past, look at your mind now. If you want to look at where you are going in the future, look at your actions now.

Several times throughout the day today, ask yourself

When I look at the state of my body and mind right now, what does that say about my past and where I have been directing my energy?

What am I doing at this very moment?

When I look at my actions now, what am I creating through this action in which I am engaging?

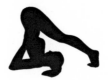

Yoga Pose for Day Eighteen

PLOW POSE (*HALASANA*)

Benefits: Relieves insomnia, calms the mind, stimulates the thyroid gland, promotes digestion, reduces stress, helpful for infertility or during menopause, and beneficial for sinusitis.

Do not do this pose if you have neck injuries or experience neck pain when coming into the pose. With your feet touching the floor overhead, the Plow Pose is considered to be an intermediate to advanced pose. It is not advisable to perform the full expression of the pose without sufficient prior experience or without the supervision of an experienced instructor.

Lie on your back with your arms alongside your body. Bend your knees into your chest. Lift your tailbone off the floor, and place your palms on your lower back. Walk your palms down toward your shoulders. Lift the tailbone toward the ceiling with the spine relatively perpendicular to the floor. Hinge at the hip joints, and slowly lower your toes to the floor beyond your head with your legs fully extended. Keeping the toes on the floor, lift your thighs and tailbone toward the ceiling. Continue to press your hands against the back torso, pushing the tailbone up toward the ceiling as you press the backs of the upper arms down into the floor. Or you can release your hands away from your back, and stretch the arms out behind you on the floor. Clasp the hands and press the arms actively down into the floor as you lift the thighs toward the ceiling.

Plow Pose is often followed by Fish Pose (see Day Seventeen), but if you are using Plow Pose to counter insomnia, then you should avoid Fish Pose because it is stimulating and will negate the sleep-inducing effect of the Plow Pose.

DRINK YOUR GREEN VEGETABLES

If you are following a 100 percent raw-food diet, even just for the next few days, incorporating more dark leafy greens will be extremely beneficial for optimizing both nutrition and cleansing. In addition to working as a strong cleansing agent on the cellular level, greens also will give you more energy and make you more alert.

In addition to the nutritive benefits of eating greens (like getting a highly absorbable form of calcium), greens also provide both fiber and chlorophyll. So eating greens cleanses your digestive tract on a daily basis. And people who have an acidic pH balance in their body could benefit from consuming up to 80 percent greens in their diet.

However, consuming a large amount of greens in salad form can be daunting. First, in order to get maximum benefit, you need to break down the leafy greens to the cellular level, which requires a lot of chewing. It can be very helpful to consume a portion of your daily greens in the form of blended soups or smoothies. One needs fewer greens in the form of green smoothies than in the form of salad because blended greens assimilate several times more thoroughly than chewed greens.

In essence, a green smoothie is a fruit smoothie with green leafy vegetables blended in. You get all the nutrition of the leafy greens, and the sweet taste of the fruit makes it extremely palatable.

If you are just starting out on green smoothies, you can begin with some of the milder green lettuces such as romaine or Bibb lettuce. Your first smoothies may be mostly fruit with just a small amount of leafy greens added in.

As you get more accustomed to the taste of the green part of the smoothie, you can increase the greens content. Ideally, you will end up with anywhere from 40 to 60 percent of your green smoothie consisting of dark leafy greens. Over time, you also can introduce more of the darker, stronger-tasting greens such as kale, collards, spinach, mustard greens, and dandelion greens.

Fresh green juices made in a juicer tend to oxidize quickly, losing their nutritive potency and taking on a bitter taste. Green smoothies, on the other hand, tend to stay bright green and taste fresh for hours if kept in a cold place. It is thought that the fiber—present in smoothies but absent in juices—prevents the mixture from oxidizing.

I strongly suggest that you try to incorporate one green smoothie into your diet every day.

If you plan on drinking green smoothies regularly, you might consider purchasing a high-quality blender such as a Vitamix, Blendtec, or K-Tec. These have powerful motors that can withstand heavy use. For now, though, you might just want to use the blender you have and see how you like incorporating green smoothies (as well as blended soups) into your daily diet.

I hope that you will join me in aspiring to awaken to the present moment and to have your thoughts and actions in the here and now create vibrant health and well-being.

RECIPES FOR DAY EIGHTEEN

Parsley-Carrot Juice

Handful of parsley

6 carrots

Juice all ingredients in a juicer, and drink immediately.

Bitter Greens and Fruit Smoothie

(Makes 1 quart)

1 small leaf aloe vera, with skin on

2 leaves chard, stems removed

1 cup chickweed

1 banana

1 peach

1 pear

Blend all ingredients together in a blender until smooth.

Raw Borscht

(Makes 3 to 4 servings)

1 cup water

1 beet, peeled

1 inch fresh ginger root, peeled

2 cloves of garlic, peeled

3 bay leaves

Blend all ingredients together, and set aside.

1 cup of water

1 carrot

1 stalk celery

1 tablespoon apple cider vinegar

2 teaspoons of raw honey or raw agave nectar

¼ cup extra-virgin olive oil

Sea salt to taste

Blend together for thirty seconds.

¼ head cabbage, grated

1 carrot, grated

½ bunch of parsley

Add grated ingredients to blended mixtures, and serve.

Spinach Salad with Cashews, Avocado, and Cranberries

1 cup baby spinach

⅓ cup cashews, raw

¼ cup dried cranberries

½ avocado, organic

1 teaspoon lime juice

Cut avocado into bite-size chunks, and sprinkle with lime juice. Toss all ingredients together.

Pumpkin-Squash Couscous

(Makes 2 servings)

For the Sauce:

1½ cups red bell pepper, chopped

¼ cup habanero pepper, chopped

2 cups yellow bell pepper, chopped

2 cups tomatoes, seeds removed, chopped

¼ cup raw agave nectar

1 shallot, chopped

½ cup extra-virgin olive oil

Sea salt

Freshly ground black pepper

Toss the pepper, agave nectar, shallot, and ¼ cup of the olive oil together in a bowl. Season with salt and pepper. Allow mixture to sit for several hours. Drain off the excess liquid. Place pepper mixture in a blender along with the remaining ¼ cup olive oil. Blend until smooth. Set aside.

For the Pumpkin-Squash Mixture:

1 shallot, minced

2 teaspoons fresh thyme

2 teaspoons ground cumin

½ teaspoon ground cinnamon

¼ cup extra-virgin olive oil

2 tablespoons almond milk (see Recipes chapter)

2 cups peeled, seeded, diced pumpkin

2 cups yellow squash, cut into half moons

Sea salt

Freshly ground black pepper

¼ cup fresh parsley, minced

¼ cup fresh cilantro, minced

Combine shallot, thyme, cumin, cinnamon, olive oil, and almond milk. Place pumpkin and squash in two separate bowls. Divide the olive oil mixture between the two bowls, toss well, and season with salt and pepper.

Allow pumpkin and squash to marinate for several hours. Combine with parsley and cilantro.

For the Couscous:

3 cups chopped jicama (one-inch cubes)

¼ cup pine nuts

½ cup dried currants

¼ cup almond oil

Coarse sea salt

Pumpkin seeds for garnish

Place jicama in food processor, and pulse several times until chopped to the size of couscous. Press between two kitchen towels or paper towels to remove excess moisture. The mixture should be dry and fluffy.

Chop pine nuts in a food processor until finely chopped. Add to the couscous along with the currants, almond oil, and salt. Combine the squash and pumpkin with the couscous. Garnish with pumpkin seeds and serve with the pepper sauce.

DAY
NINETEEN

We are not just our emotions. Our emotions come and go, but
we are always here.

—Thich Nhat Hanh

Although at times we feel ourselves controlled by our feelings, within us we possess the
calm, still, solid strength of a mountain. Our inherent stability can be a source of deep
peace for us. In our exercise for today, we dwell on our innate, inherent strength, the
mountain-solid nature of our existence.

Exercise for Day Nineteen

MOUNTAIN SOLID

Lie down in a quiet place. Take a few moments to settle into your body.
Notice the emotions that arise. Let yourself dwell in your emotions for a
few minutes, just watching the feelings as they come up.

Then bring your awareness to your breath. Take several deep, relaxed breaths. Observe the rise and fall of your abdomen and chest.
Focus on your lower abdomen, the region about two fingers' width
below the navel.

Breath slowly and fully, holding the thought:
Breathing in, I see myself as a mountain.
Breathing out, I feel solid.

Take several deep, full breaths, reciting this verse.

Reflect once again on your emotions. Observe whether your feelings may have shifted as a result of this brief breathing exercise. When
we take the time to witness our emotions over a period of time, we
realize that we are not defined by our emotions. Our emotions come
and go, but we are always here—mountain solid.

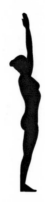

Yoga Pose for Day Nineteen

MOUNTAIN POSE (*TADASANA*)

Benefits: Improves posture and balance and strengthens the
legs, spine, and abdominal muscles.

Do not do this pose if you are light-headed or have very low blood pressure.
Stand with your feet hip width apart. Bring the weight of your pelvis back. Do
not tuck your tailbone under or flatten your lower back. Draw your shoulder
blades slightly together, and slide them down toward your waist. Observe your
breath for five to seven long, relaxed breaths.

RAW ATHLETES

I hope that you are feeling light in body and spirit as you approach the final few days of
your cleanse. Perhaps you are feeling enthused and excited about the newfound energy
and vibrancy you are experiencing by eating 100 percent raw foods. But just in case your
enthusiasm is flagging, you might be inspired to hear about some accomplished athletes
who have excelled on a raw vegan diet. These athletes believe that raw foods help to
repair the damage done by the stress of their sport and that a raw vegan diet provides
the nutrients they need to rebuild muscle tissue for increased strength and athletic performance.

Brendan Brazier

Brendan Brazier is one of only a few professional athletes in the world whose diet is
100 percent plant-based. He is a professional ironman triathlete, best-selling author on
performance nutrition, and creator of an award-winning line of whole-food nutritional
products called VEGA. Braazier is also a two-time Canadian 50-Kilometer Ultra Marathon Champion.

   Brazier's professional athletic career began in 1998. Over the course of only a few
years, his performance climbed quickly, improving each year in ironman triathlon racing. At Ironman Canada in 1999, Brazier finished twenty-first; the following year he

placed fourteenth; and then eleventh, followed up by an eighth place finish in 2002 in Ironman Utah. In 2003 and 2006, Brazier won first place in the National 50-Kilometer Ultra Marathon Championships. Other results include third place at the National Long-Course Triathlon Championships and both third and second place in consecutive years in the Royal Victoria Marathon.

Toward the end of 2003, Brazier was hit by a car while cycling and spent his recovery time writing a book that outlined the successful diet that had helped him to improve his athletic performance. The Thrive Diet quickly became a Canadian best seller. Brazier then partnered with a sports nutrition company and produced a commercial replica of the blended drink formula that he had been making for himself for fifteen years. The drink, which he called VEGA, became one of the best-selling health food products on the Canadian market and received the prestigious Nutrition Business Journal Merit Award. Brazier later launched his 100 percent raw whole-food energy bar, again a commercial replica of what he made to support his intense training.

Brazier has addressed the U.S. Congress on the subject of the significant social and economic benefits that could be achieved by improving personal health through better diet. The focus of his speech was to draw attention to the role that food plays in the prevention of most chronic diseases currently plaguing North Americans.

Tim Van Orden

In just five years, Tim Van Orden transformed himself from a sedentary couch potato suffering from severe depression and chronic fatigue syndrome into one of the world's fittest men over age forty. He attributes much of his success to a simple, plant-based diet. Creator of the Running Raw Project, this elite raw vegan athlete has consistently shattered the myths and misconceptions that surround the viability of a raw vegan diet for serious athletes. Van Orden has excelled in some of the world's most grueling sports. He is a three-time U.S. Trail Running Champion, the 2010 USA Masters Mountain Runner of the Year, and the top U.S. finisher (fourth overall) in the 2011 Stair Climbing World Championships up the Empire State Building. He has been featured in *GQ*, *The Wall Street Journal*, *VegNews*, and *The London Guardian*, as well as on the Food Network show *My Life in Food*.

For several years Van Orden meticulously tracked the effect of various training and food regimens on his athletic performance. He says, "Moving to a raw vegan diet was the best choice I've ever made as an athlete. My endurance has improved dramatically, and I recover from hard training and races in less than half the time. I've had to stop doing upper body workouts at the gym because I now build muscle *too quickly*, which slows me down as a runner. My asthma is gone, and I'm no longer troubled by joint pain."

Bob Mionske

Bob Mionske is a nationally recognized lawyer and advocate for the rights of cyclists. A former U.S. Olympic and professional cyclist, Mionske amassed a record of over 100 wins during his racing career. He represented the United States in the 1988 Olympic Games in Seoul, South Korea, where he made the winning break in the men's individual road race, finishing in fourth place. In 1990, Mionske was the U.S. National Champion in the men's road race. Mionske again made the U.S. Olympic team for the 1992 games in Barcelona, Spain, assisting teammate Lance Armstrong to a fourteenth place finish. Mionske turned professional after the 1992 games, racing for Team Saturn for one season, and then retired to become director of the team for 1993.

Mionske stopped eating meat as a teenager. Later in his life, he removed chicken and fish from his diet and describes switching to a raw vegan diet as a natural progression on the ladder of healthy eating.

James Southwood

This salvate (French kickboxing) expert has been a raw-food vegan since 2004. He needs no introduction among the martial arts crowd. He burst onto the scene in 2006 when he won his first international bout in the World Salvate Assault Championship. He also was undefeated in the British rounds for the entire year of 2006. About the raw diet, Southwood says, "Being raw is a light, clean, and pure way to live. Exercising and competing in this physical state is the only way I would choose to do it."

Scott Jurek

Scott Jurek is an accomplished ultramarathoner from Seattle, Washington. He also happens to be a proud vegan. If you are a marathon fan, you may have heard of the 2008 Spartathlon, a 246-kilometer (153-mile) historic ultramarathon course between the historic cities of Athens and Sparta in Greece. Jurek won that race, along with the two other races before that. Jurek currently holding some of the best times in race history.

Jurek's stamina, endurance, and strength are sustained by an all-vegan diet. Often his regular, effortless twenty-five-mile run is simply a warm-up to his daily training. Jurek's boundless energy more than speaks for itself. He says that meeting his extremely high daily calorie requirement of 5,000 to 8,000 calories is not so much a matter of what you eat but more about how much you eat. His 1,000-calorie smoothies made from fresh oils, bananas, blueberries, almonds, coconut, dates, and brown rice protein powder are a calorie supplement to his ample meals of greens, herbs, vegetables, miso, tofu, shallots, lemons, and many more.

If you are thinking about adopting a vegetarian, vegan, or raw-food vegan diet, know that it is an achievable lifestyle, even if you expend many calories through intensive exercise. You simply require a readiness to change and the determination to succeed.

RECIPES FOR DAY NINETEEN

Cantaloupe Juice

Cut a cantaloupe into strips, and keep the rind intact.
Juice the cantaloupe in a juicer, and drink immediately.

Summer Green Smoothie

2 leaves chard, stems removed

2 stalks celery

½ bunch fresh parsley

3 apricots

2 peaches

½ vanilla bean

Blend all ingredients together in a blender until smooth.

Cucumber-Dill Soup

(Makes 2 servings)

1 cucumber

½ cup fresh dill

1 small avocado

2 leaves dinosaur kale, stems removed

1 stalk celery

2 tablespoons lime juice

1 clove garlic

Blend all ingredients in a blender or food processor to desired consistency.

Lavender-Berry Salad

1 cup baby greens

1 tomato, sliced

2 ripe peaches, sliced

½ cup strawberries, sliced

½ cup blueberries

½ cup microgreens

Combine all ingredients, and toss gently.

For the Lavender Dressing:

6 tablespoons olive oil

2 tablespoons apple cider vinegar

1 tablespoon lemon juice

2 tablespoons raw honey

1 teaspoon Dijon mustard

1 teaspoon dried lavender flowers, ground or whole

Whisk all the ingredients together, and allow to sit for about thirty minutes. Pour over the salad, toss, and serve.

* *

Summer Rolls with Green Papaya

(Makes 4 to 6 rolls)

For the Filling:

½ cup green papaya or green mango, peeled and julienned

½ cup young coconut meat, julienned

½ large carrot, julienned

2 radishes, finely julienned

2 tablespoons julienned ginger

2 tablespoons Nama Shoyu soy sauce

2 tablespoons mirin—optional

2 tablespoons lime juice

1 tablespoon raw agave nectar

½ tablespoon sesame oil

½ long red chili pepper, seeded and minced

Sea salt

Freshly ground black pepper

Combine green papaya (or mango), coconut meat, carrots, radishes, and ginger in a bowl and set aside.

Whisk together the Nama Shoyu, raw agave nectar, lime juice, mirin, sesame oil, and chili pepper. Pour over the papaya mixture, and toss gently. Allow to marinate for at least thirty minutes. Drain mixture before assembling the rolls.

For the Dipping Sauce:

1 red bell pepper

1 red chili pepper, chopped with seeds

½ cup young coconut meat

2 tablespoons coconut water

Sea salt

Freshly ground black pepper to taste

Blend the bell pepper and the red chili pepper along with the coconut meat in a blender until smooth. Add coconut water as needed. Season with salt and pepper, and set aside.

For the Assembly:

1 large daikon radish or 3 medium cucumbers, peeled

½ cup finely chopped almonds

1 tablespoon almond oil

1 ripe avocado, sliced

1 handful basil leaves

1 handful raw sunflower seeds

2 tablespoons sesame seeds (black or white)

Using a sharp knife or a mandoline, cut the daikon or the cucumber into thin slices about four inches long. Use the widest slices for the assembly.

Toss the almonds with the oil, and set aside.

Lay out a sheet of daikon or cucumber or use several overlapping slices. Place a small handful of the filling lengthwise on the slices, and top with almonds, avocado slices, basil leaves, and sprouts. Allow the leafy ends to extend beyond the ends of the wrapper. Carefully roll tightly.

Sprinkle the rolls with sesame seeds, and serve with the dipping sauce.

DAY TWENTY

The most important thing is remembering the most important thing.

—Anonymous

Today's message is for the person who has at one time or another felt as though she has fallen short. It is for the person who sometimes believes that he has missed the mark and does not quite measure up, the person who often tells herself that she is somehow wrong, whose sense of self is defined by a basic inadequacy. In short, today's message is probably for each and every one of us.

Perhaps our most difficult and yet most pervasive suffering is caused by our feelings of inadequacy. Tara Brach calls this the "trance of unworthiness"—a waking dream in which, ultimately, no matter what we achieve, we still feel that we are fundamentally not good enough. The belief in our deficiency, the sense that we are failing or are going to fail, and our need to hide it from others populate our life with fear and anxiety.

If we have a worthwhile quest, it might be to seek the freedom that comes with kindness and true appreciation of ourselves and others. Seng-tsan, the renowned seventh-century Zen master, taught that true freedom is being "without anxiety about imperfections." This means accepting our human existence and all of life just as it is. Imperfection is not our unique, personal problem. Imperfection is rather a natural, integral part of our existence. If we can relax about our imperfections, even get to a place where we welcome them, then we can stop living from fear. We can let go of our relentless pursuit of self-improvement. Then we can find true freedom in the beautifully, perfectly imperfect moments of life.

Of course, self-love and self-esteem have a tremendous impact on our personal health. If we care for ourselves, we will want to make good choices about how we eat, how we exercise, and how we use our time. Hopefully, we will resist the tendency to have those choices be driven by a desire to punish ourselves for our perceived deficiencies. Ideally, our lifestyle choices will be motivated by a wish to nurture and care for ourselves as though we were our own best friend.

More important, self-compassion is an absolute prerequisite to loving others. If we want to love without holding back, and if we want to be truly free, we must get there by accepting and appreciating ourselves in the moment, just as we are.

The exercise for today seeks to develop skills to stay with your thoughts and feelings about yourself. "The only way that you'll actually wake up and have some freedom is if you have the capacity and courage to stay with the vulnerability and the discomfort" (Tara Brach).

Practice coming alongside yourself like a true, loving friend. Seek to meet whatever is there with kindness and compassion, and gain more of the freedom it takes to love yourself and others fully.

Exercise for Day Twenty

BECOMING YOUR FRIEND

Sit or lie down in a quiet place. Tune into the natural rhythm of your breath. Allow yourself to relax.

Ask yourself

What is happening inside me right now?
What is the quality of my thoughts and feelings?
Where do I feel some pain or discomfort, physically or emotionally?

Let yourself stay present to the vulnerability that comes with discomfort.

Now imagine someone who truly loves you beholding your suffering and sending you compassion. Sense that person's love for you filling your heart.

You might choose to pause throughout your day today to notice where you feel pain and imagine the love of a friend filling you with care and healing. Over time and with practice, we become that friend to ourselves.

Yoga Pose for Day Twenty

HEAD-OF-THE-KNEE POSE
(*JANU SIRSASANA*)

Benefits: Stretches the hamstrings and lengthens the spine, opens the muscles across the lower spine, and aids digestion.

Do not do this pose if you have diagnosed disk disease in your lower back. Practice with caution if you have knee pain or a knee injury. Sit with your legs extended out in front of you. Bend your right knee in toward your chest, and let the right knee fall out to the right. Bring the sole of your right foot to your right inner thigh. Ideally, your right shin will be perpendicular to your left leg. Tilt your pelvis slightly forward, turn your chest toward your left knee, and extend your chest forward toward your left shin. Drop your head and lengthen your spine out over your left leg. Take five to ten deep breaths, and change sides.

A daily meditation practice is so very helpful for your inner peace and self-understanding. I cannot emphasize this enough. Take just five minutes each day to quiet yourself and become intimate with your experience. If you can make time for this short meditation in the morning, I promise you that it will create more moments of presence and freedom throughout your day.

If you take away nothing else from this cleanse, a regular meditation practice is the single most valuable piece I can recommend. Meditation has the power to transform your life in the most profound of ways. I do not know of a better gift to your spirit.

Tomorrow marks the last day of your cleanse. You may be wondering about making the transition back to a sustainable way of eating and moving through your days. So today is a good time to consider your aspirations beyond the cleanse.

How would you like to continue to incorporate some of the changes you made during these past three weeks into your daily life going forward? What do you think will be the best way for you to eat for your body and lifestyle? There is a broad spectrum here, from simply eating less processed foods to adopting a 100 percent raw vegan diet, with many choices in between. Will you do without dairy? eggs? meat? How much cooked food seems ideal to you? Will you continue to make fresh fruit and vegetable juices and smoothies on a daily basis? Would you like to stay with eating only fresh fruits until noon and then eating from "light to heavy" for the remainder of the day, slowing down at sunset to give your digestive system a longer rest? What about refined sugar and caffeine?

And how about the other habits you my have cultivated in recent weeks? Can you commit to a daily yoga practice, even if on some days this simply means a brief ten- to fifteen-minute home practice on your own? Would you like to cultivate a regular meditation routine, setting aside just five minutes each day (preferably first thing in the morning) to be quiet and still? What about getting outdoors on a daily basis to dwell on the beauty of nature?

How much would you like to unplug from the media that can camouflage your authentic experience of life? Can you be less tied to your cell phone and computer and make more mindful choices about music, films, the Internet, and other reading material?

Take a few minutes today to reflect on your big-picture intentions: Where would you like to be in terms of your diet and lifestyle habits?

"The most important thing is remembering the most important thing." Which positive changes from our cleanse can you sustain into the long term, and what will serve you best? I suggest writing your aspirations down. In this way, you can read them regularly to stay inspired and on track or revise them from time to time as your interests and needs change in the future.

In terms of food, I suggest that you work backwards in introducing food groups back into your diet. In other words, go back out the same way you came in. If you are now eating 100 percent raw foods, then the first thing to reintroduce would be some lightly cooked vegetables.

Allow yourself a few days to adjust to that. If you like, you then can reintroduce some cooked whole grains, again giving yourself a few days or even a few weeks to acclimate to these denser foods.

If you want to include animal products in your diet going forward, then you can add some eggs and dairy products first and then perhaps add some lighter animal protein such as fish and chicken. It will be important to make this an incremental process and to afford adequate time for your system to accommodate these foods because they will be much more difficult to process.

Finally, you may choose to return to eating some foods containing sugar and flour, such as bread, pasta, pastries, cookies, and cakes, as well as chocolate and coffee, but I encourage you to be mindful of how your body reacts to all these food groups and to assess whether they will serve you well in the long term.

A light, highly cleansing diet is wonderful in terms of gaining physical energy, emotional awareness, and spiritual clarity. But it also can be challenging to sustain that level of intensity in your daily life. The degree to which you want to commit to a healthier lifestyle into the future is entirely personal. While I believe that a whole foods–based diet comprised primarily of raw fruits and vegetables is ideal, you will need to find the balance that meets your own unique needs and beliefs. I invite you to hold yourself lightly and follow a path of moderation that makes allowances for small indulgences from time to time. I believe that restricting ourselves with food can be far more toxic than eating a little bit of less-than-healthy fare every once in a while. Please try to keep your eating habits in perspective and be gentle with yourself. Focus on the positive effects of nourishing yourself with healthy, vibrant, whole foods rather than on limiting or restricting yourself. "The most important thing is remembering the most important thing."

Please contact me through www.gratitudeyoga.org if I can support you in determining and maintaining diet and lifestyle habits that move you toward health, wholeness, and inner peace.

RECIPES FOR DAY TWENTY

Apple-Grape Juice

2 apples
1 large bunch of grapes
1 slice lemon with peel
Juice all ingredients in a juicer, and drink immediately.

Cucumber–Dandelion Green Smoothie

½ bunch dandelion greens
1 medium cucumber
1½ cups water
Blend all ingredients together in a blender until smooth.

Gazpacho

(Makes 2 servings)

1 leaf kale, finely chopped

3 tablespoons fresh basil, chopped

3 tablespoons fresh cilantro, chopped

1 tomato, diced

½ stalk celery, diced

½ red bell pepper, diced

½ avocado

2 tablespoons lime juice

2 tablespoons extra-virgin olive oil

⅓ cup water

Pulse all ingredients in a food processor until combined but still chunky. Allow to sit for thirty minutes or longer before serving.

Ginger-Carrot Coleslaw

(Makes 2 servings)

2 carrots, grated

1 cup red cabbage, shredded

½ cup raisins

2 tablespoons sunflower seeds

2 teaspoons pumpkin seeds

Toss all ingredients together until combined.

For the Dressing:

1 teaspoon raw honey

1 tablespoon lemon juice

2 teaspoons grated ginger

2 tablespoons cold-pressed oil of your choice

Dash of sea salt

Dissolve the honey in the lemon juice. Add the remaining ingredients. Pour over the salad, and toss. Allow salad to marinate for about fifteen to thirty minutes.

* *

Spring Rolls and Raw Teriyaki Sauce

(Makes 5 servings)

For the Teriyaki Sauce:

½ cup Nama Shoyu soy sauce

½ cup pure maple syrup

½ teaspoon ginger, whole

½ clove garlic

1 drizzle sesame oil

Blend all the ingredients, and use as a dipping sauce.

For the Spring Rolls:

½ red bell pepper, julienned

½ large carrot, julienned

½ cup whole cilantro leaves

¼ cup fresh mint leaves, chopped

½ cup whole basil leaves

5 whole red or green cabbage leaves

Place bell pepper, carrots, cilantro, mint, and basil inside
a cabbage leaf. Roll the cabbage leaf, and dip in teriyaki
sauce.

* *

DAY
TWENTY-ONE

> . . . [W]e can put our trust in the power of self-healing, self-
> understanding, and loving within us. We call this the island
> within ourselves in which we can take refuge. It is an island of
> peace, confidence, solidity, love, and freedom.
>
> —*Thich Nhat Hanh*

Today concludes your twenty-one-day cleanse. Whether you implemented all the sug-
gestions about diet and lifestyle or made just few tiny tweaks, your desire to be receptive
to change reveals a bigger, deeper desire to awaken to your true potential, which is to
live meaningfully and with joy. That desire to be awake and alive is an innate quality for
which you should be immensely grateful. It tells you that you are already on the path.

A willingness to trust in the power of self-healing while pursuing self-understanding and cultivating the seeds of love and compassion toward yourself is the critical first
step in charting your course. Along the way, at any given moment, you can come home
to the here and now and take refuge in the island within yourself—an island of peace,
confidence, solidity, love, and freedom.

As you know, your aspiration to awaken is not simply a wish to attain peace and
freedom for yourself. It is a much broader intention that embraces others. You see this
play out in practical terms in your life. When you are calm and at ease, when you act
out of kindness, it almost always influences those around you. In a family, if there is one
person who practices mindfulness, the entire family will be more mindful. If in a yoga
class there is one person who moves with mindfulness and awareness, the rest of the
class is inspired by that person's authentic presence. If in our places of work we can treat
others with calm gentleness, it is sure to permeate the environment. Thich Nhat Hanh
uses a wonderful metaphor:

> We are like a boat crossing the ocean. If the boat encounters
> a storm and everyone panics, the boat turns over. If there is
> one person in the boat who can remain calm, that person can
> inspire others to be calm. Who is that person who can stay
> calm? Each of us is that person. We count on each other.

We count on each other. There is grace and beauty in that.

I have saved my favorite practice, Tonglin, for last. *Tonglin* is a Tibetan word meaning "giving and taking" or "sending and receiving." In this ancient Tibetan Buddhist
practice, one visualizes taking onto oneself the suffering of others on the in breath and
on the out breath giving happiness and success to all sentient beings. It is a potent training in altruism. It is my hope that it may become a more frequent practice for you.

SENDING AND RECEIVING (TONGLIN)

Sit comfortably in a peaceful place. Settle into your body, and take several full, calming breaths.

Call to mind a person for whom you care deeply, a person whose well-being you wish for. With your exhalation, send out toward that person whatever goodness you have in your life: health, joy, comfort, security, love. Do this for several minutes, sending out goodness on your out breaths.

Next, as you inhale, envision taking in all the negativity that person experiences: his or her fear, confusion, limitations, whatever brings that person suffering. Let the embodiment of that person's suffering rest on you as you inhale. With your exhalations, continue to send out goodness toward that individual.

Spend several minutes working with the breath in this way—inhaling suffering, exhaling goodness—as if a bright light were going out with your breath toward the person you have chosen.

Please note that this practice requires confidence in your ability to accommodate another person's suffering. With the incoming breath, we try to allow the embodiment of suffering to come toward us, and we let ourselves gladly take it in. However, the receiving of another's suffering can be extremely challenging, even overwhelming. If you feel overcome by the difficulty of taking in suffering, please omit that part of the practice and concentrate on sending out goodness with your out breath. You can revisit the "receiving" part of the practice in the future.

The Dalai Lama, who practices Tonglin every day, has said of this technique: "Whether this meditation really helps others or not, it gives me peace of mind. Then I can be more effective, and the benefit is immense."

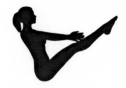

Yoga Pose for Day Twenty-One
BOAT POSE (*NAVASANA*)
Benefits: Strengthens the abdominal muscles and the spine
and improves digestion.

Do not do this pose if you have neck pain or injury or if you feel pain in the lower back. Sit on the floor with your legs straight in front of you. Place your palms on the floor behind your hips with your fingers pointing toward your feet. Lift the chest, and lean back slightly. Maintain length in your spine. Resist the temptation to round the back.

Bend your knees into your chest. Lift your feet so that your thighs are at a sixty-degree angle to the floor. Gradually straighten your knees. Raise the tips of your toes slightly above eye level. If this isn't possible, then keep your knees bent, perhaps lifting the shins parallel to the floor. You may either hold onto the backs of your knees or reach your arms out alongside your legs. Hold this pose for one or two breaths, eventually extending your time in the pose to several minutes.

RECIPES FOR DAY TWENTY-ONE

Liver Cleanse Juice

2–3 carrots
½ beet
Juice all ingredients in a juicer, and drink immediately.

Banana-Mango Green Smoothie

(Makes 1 quart)

¼ head romaine lettuce
1 ripe banana, peeled and frozen
1 orange, peeled, seeds removed

½ mango

1 cup water

Blend all ingredients together in a blender until smooth.

* *

Butternut-Leek Soup

(Makes 3 to 4 servings)

1 small, fresh leek

1 bunch celery

½ butternut squash, peeled and deseeded

1 small avocado

2 tablespoons tahini

4 tablespoons flaxseed oil or olive oil

1 teaspoon sea salt

3 tablespoons chives, minced

Freshly ground black pepper to taste

Juice the leeks and the celery in a juicer. Shred the squash in a food processor. Blend the celery-leek juice in a blender with the shredded squash. Add water to reach desired consistency. Garnish with minced chives.

* *

Cinnamon Spice Salad

(Makes 2 servings)

½ pound romaine or baby lettuce, chopped

1 cup cherry or grape tomatoes, sliced in half

1 teaspoon cinnamon

1 teaspoon ground cloves

1 clove garlic, chopped

1 teaspoon fresh oregano, chopped

1 teaspoon fresh thyme, chopped

2 tablespoons fresh lemon juice

Raw honey or raw agave nectar to taste

4 raw olives, chopped

Sea salt and freshly ground black pepper to taste

Combine all the ingredients, and toss well.

* *

Broccoli in Hoisin Sauce with Raw Rice

(Makes 1 to 2 servings)

5 cups small broccoli florets

2 tablespoons lemon juice

3 tablespoons olive oil

1 tablespoon tamari

Mix all ingredients together until the broccoli becomes softer. Allow to marinate for about an hour.

For the Hoisin Sauce:

¼ cup tahini

1 teaspoon lemon juice

1 teaspoon yacon syrup or agave nectar

1 teaspoon apple cider vinegar

3 teaspoons tamari

½ clove garlic

½ small chili pepper, deseeded

½-cm cube fresh ginger

Blend all ingredients in a high-speed blender until smooth.

Pour sauce over marinated broccoli, and toss well. Serve with Parsnip Rice (see below).

For the Parsnip Rice:

1½ cups peeled, chopped parsnips

1½ tablespoons pine nuts

1 tablespoon macadamia nuts

1 tablespoon light miso

1 tablespoon cold-pressed sesame oil

3 spring onions, finely chopped

Process all ingredients except the spring onions in a food processor until fluffy and rice-like. Stir in the chopped spring onions and serve.

Recipes

JUICES/SMOOTHIES/NUT MILKS/TEAS

Fortifying Juice

6 oz carrot juice

1 oz beet juice

1 oz parsley or watercress juice

Juice all ingredients in a juicer, and drink immediately.

Calming Cocktail

5 oz carrot juice

3 oz celery juice

Juice all ingredients in a juicer, and drink immediately.

Lemon-Lime Ginger Ale

Handful of grapes

1 apple, cored and sliced

½ inch fresh ginger (less if you find the taste too strong)

½ lime

¼ lemon

Sparkling mineral water

Remove the grapes from the stem. Juice the apple and ginger together, and then juice the rest of the fruit. Pour the juice into a large glass, fill to the top with sparkling water, and serve with ice.

* *

Sparkling Tropical Fruit Juice

1 kiwi, peeled
1 orange, peeled and sectioned
½ mango, peeled and sliced
Sparkling mineral water
Juice all ingredients in a juicer, and drink immediately.

* *

Potassium Drink

4 medium carrots, greens removed
1 stalk celery
1 apple
Handful of fresh parsley
Handful of fresh spinach
½ lemon, peeled—optional
Juice all ingredients in a juicer, and drink immediately.

* *

Carrot-Apple Juice

6 carrots
2 apples
Juice all ingredients in a juicer, and drink immediately.

* *

Apple-Kale-Lemon Juice

4 apples
Juice of ½ lemon
5 leaves kale
2 cups water
Juice all ingredients in a juicer, and drink immediately.

* *

Pear-Kale-Mint Juice

4 ripe pears
5 leaves kale

½ bunch mint

2 cups water

Juice all ingredients in a juicer, and drink immediately.

* *

Cucumber-Celery Juice

3–4 stalks celery

½ cucumber

Juice all ingredients in a juicer, and drink immediately.

* *

Fennel Juice

½ small fennel bulb

1 apple

2 carrots

¼ beetroot

Juice all ingredients in a juicer, and drink immediately.

* *

Mixed Vegetable Juice

1 kale leaf

1 collard leaf

Small handful of parsley

1 stalk celery

1 carrot, greens removed

½ red pepper

1 tomato

1 broccoli floret

Celery stalk for garnish

Juice leaves and parsley and then the celery and carrot. Follow with red pepper, tomato, and broccoli. Garnish with celery stalk.

* *

Sunshine Juice

4 Granny Smith or Gravenstein apples

2 inches fresh ginger, peeled

1 Meyer lemon, peeled

4 oz water to dilute

Juice all ingredients in a juicer, and drink immediately.

· ·

Ginger-Grape Juice

2 cups red grapes

2 inches fresh ginger, peeled

1 Meyer lemon, peeled

½ cup water—optional

Juice all ingredients in a juicer, and drink immediately.

· ·

Refreshing Ginger Fruit Juice

2 nectarines or peaches

½ cantaloupe

2 apples

1-inch ginger claw

2 tablespoons ground flax seeds

Juice all ingredients in a juicer. Add 1 cup of ice cubes, and blend in a blender until smooth.

· ·

Carrot-Apple Juice

6 carrots

2 apples

Juice all ingredients in a juicer, and drink immediately.

· ·

Liver Cleanse Juice

2–3 carrots

½ beet

Juice all ingredients in a juicer, and drink immediately.

· ·

Digestive Aid Juice

1 pineapple

Remove top but keep skin intact. Juice pineapple in a juicer, and drink immediately.

Apple-Pear Juice

2 apples

1 pear

Juice all ingredients in a juicer, and drink immediately.

Spinach-Carrot Juice

Handful of spinach

6 carrots

Juice all ingredients in a juicer, and drink immediately.

Apple-Grape Juice

2 apples

1 large bunch of grapes

1 slice lemon with peel

Juice all ingredients in a juicer, and drink immediately.

Carrot-Cucumber-Beet Juice

4 carrots

½ cucumber

1 beet

Juice all ingredients in a juicer, and drink immediately.

Rejuvenating Juice

Handful of parsley

3 carrots

2 stalks celery

2 cloves garlic

Juice all ingredients in a juicer, and drink immediately.

Cantaloupe Juice

1 cantaloupe

Cut cantaloupe into strips, and keep rind intact. Juice cantaloupe in a juicer, and drink immediately.

Apple-Celery Juice

1 stalk celery

2 apples

Juice all ingredients in a juicer, and drink immediately.

Apple-Strawberry Juice

2 apples

4–6 strawberries

Juice all ingredients in a juicer, and drink immediately.

Parsley-Carrot Juice

Handful of parsley

6 carrots

Juice all ingredients in a juicer, and drink immediately.

Watermelon Juice

½ small watermelon
Cut melon into strips, and keep rind intact. Juice watermelon in a juicer, and drink immediately.

Passion Juice

4 strawberries
½ pineapple
1 bunch black grapes
Juice all ingredients in a juicer, and drink immediately.

Morning Cleanse Juice

1 apple
1 grapefruit (peeled)
Juice all ingredients in a juicer, and drink immediately.

Citrus Cleansing Juice

¼ lemon with peel
½ grapefruit (peeled)
2 oranges (peeled)
Juice all ingredients in a juicer, and drink immediately.

Alkalizing Juice

¼ head cabbage, red or green
3 stalks celery
Juice all ingredients in a juicer, and drink immediately.

SMOOTHIES

Electrolyte Lemonade

½ cup raw agave nectar or raw honey

2 tablespoons coconut butter, blended with about ½ cup warm water

¼ cup peeled fresh ginger

¼ teaspoon turmeric, blended with ½ cup water

2 apples, cored and peeled

2 lemons, partially peeled (leave white pith on if possible)

½ teaspoon sun-dried sea salt

1–2 tablespoons flax meal to taste

Blend all ingredients together in a blender until smooth.

Red Leaf and Basil Green Smoothie

(Makes 1 quart)

6 leaves red leaf lettuce

¼ bunch fresh basil

½ lime, juiced

½ red onion

2 stalks celery

¼ avocado

2 cups water

Blend all ingredients together in a blender until smooth.

Banana-Mango Green Smoothie

(Makes 1 quart)

¼ head romaine lettuce

1 ripe banana, peeled and frozen

1 orange, peeled, seeds removed

½ mango

1 cup water

Blend all ingredients together in a blender until smooth.

Tropical Green Smoothie

(Makes 1 quart)

1 young coconut, meat and water
3 leaves kale, stems removed
1 nectarine
1 peach
½ mango
Blend all ingredients together in a blender until smooth.

Detoxifying Green Smoothie

(Makes 1 quart)

½ bunch cilantro
1 cup stinging nettles
½ bunch fresh parsley
2 stalks celery
2 tablespoons lemon juice
1 mango
Blend all ingredients together in a blender until smooth.

Super Green Smoothie

(Makes 1 quart)

2 leaves kale, stems removed
2 leaves chard, stems removed
¼ cup fresh parsley
1 small leaf aloe vera
¼ cup dandelion greens
1 pear
1 banana
1½ cups water
Blend all ingredients together in a blender until smooth.

Cucumber–Dandelion Green Smoothie

½ bunch dandelion greens

1 medium cucumber

1½ cups water

Blend all ingredients together in a blender until smooth.

Watermelon-Lime Smoothie

(Makes 1 quart)

½ small watermelon

2 limes, juiced

Blend all ingredients together in a blender until smooth.

Revitalizing Green Smoothie

(Makes 1 quart)

3 young grape leaves (They contain resveratrol, which triggers longevity genes.)

2 leaves dinosaur kale, stems removed

1 mango

1 cup strawberries

1 cup orange juice

Blend all ingredients together in a blender until smooth.

Summer Green Smoothie

2 leaves chard, stems removed

2 stalks celery

½ bunch fresh parsley

3 apricots

2 peaches

½ vanilla bean

Blend all ingredients together in a blender until smooth.

Bitter Greens and Fruit Smoothie

(Makes 1 quart)

1 small leaf aloe vera, skin on

2 leaves chard, stems removed

1 cup chickweed

1 banana

1 peach

1 pear

Blend all ingredients together in a blender until smooth.

Wild Lettuce Smoothie

(Makes 1 quart)

1½ cups edible wild lettuce

1 ripe pear

½ cup blueberries

1 cup water

Blend all ingredients together in a blender until smooth.

Pear Smoothie

(Makes 1 quart)

1 d'Anjou pear

3 leaves purple kale, stems removed

1 small leaf aloe vera, skin on

1 banana

Blend all ingredients together in a blender until smooth.

Kale-Tomato-Basil Green Smoothie

(Makes 1 quart)

5 leaves kale, stems removed

½ bunch fresh basil

½ lime, juiced

3 cloves garlic—optional

¼ cup sun-dried tomatoes

2 cups water

Blend all ingredients together in a blender until smooth.

* *

Raspberry-Pear Green Smoothie

(Makes 1 quart)

2 Bosc pears

Handful of raspberries

4–5 leaves kale, stems removed

2 cups water

Blend all ingredients together in a blender until smooth.

* *

Berry-Banana Smoothie

2 cups fresh blueberries, raspberries, or strawberries

1 banana

1 orange

Blend all ingredients together in a blender until smooth.

* *

Watermelon-Spinach Smoothie

½ small seeded watermelon, including the peel

10 strawberries

1 bunch spinach

1 cup water

Blend all ingredients together in a blender until smooth.

* *

Mango-Kale Smoothie

(Makes 1 quart)

1 mango

1 cup kale

1 cup water

Blend all ingredients together in a blender until smooth.

* *

Energizing Smoothie

(Makes 2 quarts)

2 cups green or red seedless grapes

3 golden kiwis, peeled

1 ripe orange, peeled, seeds removed

1 small leaf of aloe vera, with skin on

5 leaves red leaf lettuce

2 cups water

Blend all ingredients together in a blender until smooth.

Wake-up Smoothie

(Makes 2 quarts)

½ bunch dandelion greens

2 stalks celery

½ inch fresh ginger root

2 peaches

½ pineapple

Blend all ingredients together in a blender until smooth.

Parsley Smoothie

(Makes 2 quarts)

1 bunch fresh parsley

1 cucumber, peeled

1 Fuji apple

1 ripe banana

1–2 cups water

Blend all ingredients together in a blender until smooth.

Super Green Smoothie

¾ pound oranges, grapes, strawberries, or other moist fruit

½ pound figs, apples, blueberries, or other fruit

1 tablespoon flax or soaked chia seed—optional

½ bunch flat leaf parsley, cilantro, or other herb

1 bunch kale, collards, bok choy, spinach, or romaine

1-2 ripe bananas

1 tablespoon spirulina or chlorella—optional

Add the first five ingredients and blend until smooth. Then add the rest and blend just until thoroughly mixed. Try to keep your blending time under one minute to reduce the chance of oxidation.

You may need to add some water to thin this out a bit depending on which fruits and vegetables you use. Some have higher water content than others. I like to have my Super Green Smoothie on the thick side because it seems more satisfying in the long term.

* *

Dark Green Smoothie

(Makes 1 quart)

½ bunch dandelion greens

2 Roma tomatoes

1½ cups water

Blend all ingredients together in a blender until smooth.

* *

Kale Green Smoothie

(Makes 2 servings)

1 ripe banana

½ cup raspberries

½ cup blueberries

3 baby carrots or ½ regular carrot

2-3 large dark green leafy kale leaves, with stalks

Handful of cruciferous greens (broccoli greens, cauliflower greens, cabbage greens, etc.)

2 cups water

2 tablespoons golden flax seeds

Blend all ingredients together in a blender until smooth.

* *

Blueberry Smoothie

(Makes 1 quart)

1 stalk celery

2 cups fresh blueberries

1 banana

2 cups water

Blend all ingredients together in blender until smooth.

Kale Smoothie

(Makes 1 quart)

5 leaves kale, stems removed

¼ avocado

3 cloves garlic

Juice of ½ lime

2 cups water

Sea salt to taste

2 Roma tomatoes

Blend all ingredients together in blender until smooth.

Pyncnogenol Passion Smoothie

1 cascade of red or black grapes, preferably with seeds

1 cup cherries, pitted and frozen

½ cup Manuka or Thompson raisins, soaked one hour in ½ cup water, reserve the soak water

½ avocado

2 cups fresh apple juice

2 tablespoons flax seed oil—optional

Pluck grapes from stem, and freeze or use at room temperature. Blend all ingredients together in a blender until smooth, about two minutes. Make sure that the seeds are ground completely. Spoon into sorbet glasses.

Strawberry-Banana-Romaine Smoothie

1 cup strawberries

2 bananas

½ bunch romaine

2 cups water

Blend all ingredients together in a blender until smooth.

NUT MILKS

Almond Milk

1 cup raw almonds, soaked four or more hours

3–6 cups charged water

3 tablespoons raw honey or raw agave nectar or stevia to taste

Pinch of Celtic sea salt

Blend all ingredients together in blender until creamy and smooth. Add water and strain to achieve a thinner consistency. If you add less water, you will have a thick "whipped cream" consistency. Store covered in the refrigerator. Keeps for several days.

Sunflower Sesame Milk

½ cup raw sunflower seeds, soaked one hour, drained, and rinsed

½ cup raw sesame seeds, ground to a meal in coffee grinder or food processor

3 cups water

2 tablespoons raw honey or 1 tablespoon liquid stevia

Sea salt to taste

Soak sunflower seeds for one hour, drain, and rinse. Grind sesame seeds in coffee grinder or food processor. Combine all ingredients together in a blender, and blend well on high for several minutes until liquefied. Strain if desired.

Macadamia Nut Milk

5 cups water

1 cup raw macadamia nuts

1 tablespoon raw honey, raw agave nectar, or maple syrup

Sea salt to taste

Put all ingredients into blender and let sit with lid on for ten minutes to soften the nuts. Blend well on high speed for up to one minute. Make this recipe with less water to create a nut creme.

TEAS

Inner Beauty Herbal Tea

1 cup dried peppermint

½ cup dried oat straw

½ cup dried alfalfa

½ cup dried sage

Combine all herbs, mix together well, and store in an air-tight container. Cover and steep 1 teaspoon of the herbal tea blend in one cup of hot water for fifteen to twenty minutes. Strain and drink warm or cool. You also may cover and steep 4 teaspoons of the herbal tea blend in 4 cups of hot water for twenty minutes, strain into a thermos, and drink throughout the day.

Peppermint aids digestion, oat straw is rich in silica, alfalfa contains many vitamins and minerals, especially potassium and iron, and sage helps to eliminate mucus in the respiratory passages and stomach.

Inner Beauty Herbal Tea with Chaparral

2 tablespoons Inner Beauty Herbal Tea (see recipe above)

2 teaspoons dried chaparral herb

6 cups hot water

Cover and steep for one hour. Drink throughout the day.

Chaparral protects against infection and promotes the elimination of toxins through the kidneys, lymph, and blood. It is a powerful herb used specifically for cleansing. It is not a good idea to use it every day. You may want to wait until week 3 of our cleanse to use chaparral.

SALAD DRESSINGS

Liquid Gold Elixir Salad Dressing

(Makes 2 cups)

1 cup fresh lemon juice

1 whole clove garlic

1-2 tablespoons minced ginger

2 tablespoons Nama Shoyu soy sauce

2 heaping tablespoons raw honey or agave syrup

¾ cup cold-pressed olive oil

Place all the ingredients except the oil in a blender. Begin blending at normal speed. Gradually pour in the oil and blend until smooth. Lasts one week in the refrigerator.

Raw Tahini Dressing

(Makes 2 cups)

1 cup raw tahini

¼ teaspoon cumin

2 tablespoons apple juice

1 clove garlic

1 tablespoon Nama Shoyu soy sauce

1 tablespoon lemon juice

1 tablespoon agave syrup

¼ cup water or apple cider vinegar

Blend all ingredients except water in a blender until smooth. This mixture thickens in the refrigerator. Add the water to dilute before serving.

Sweet Miso Dressing

(Makes 1½ cups)

2 tablespoons extra-virgin olive oil

½ clove garlic, chopped

2 medium stalks celery, cut into thirds

¼ cup water

2 tablespoons freshly squeezed lemon juice

2 tablespoons Nama Shoyu soy sauce

1 tablespoon white miso

2 organic unsulfured dates

Blend all the ingredients in a blender until smooth. This is a neutral dressing and can be used as a dip if you use less water for a thicker consistency. Keeps in the refrigerator for about ten days.

Asian Dressing

(Makes ½ cup)

2 tablespoons raw tahini

1 clove garlic, chopped

1 inch fresh ginger, chopped

1 lemon, juiced

2 tablespoons raw honey or raw agave syrup

1 teaspoon sesame oil

3 tablespoons Nama Shoyu soy sauce

Blend all the ingredients in a blender until smooth.

Raw Ranch Dressing

(Makes 2 cups)

½ cup fresh lemon juice

1 tablespoon sea salt

1 tablespoon dried rosemary

1 tablespoon dried oregano

1 tablespoon dried sage

1 cup whole macadamia nuts

⅓ cup extra-virgin olive oil—optional

Blend all the ingredients in a blender until smooth.

* * *

Carrot-Ginger Dressing

(Makes 4 cups)

1 cup baby carrots

1–2 tablespoons fresh ginger

2 tablespoons raw honey or raw agave syrup

⅓ cup apple cider vinegar

½ cup water

1 clove garlic

¼ cup flax seed oil

1 tablespoon sesame oil

Cumin, coriander, or curry spice to taste

Blend all the ingredients in a blender until smooth. Keeps in the refrigerator for two weeks.

* * *

Tahini Tamari Dressing

(Makes 1 cup)

2 tablespoons olive oil or a mixture of 1 tablespoon olive oil and 1 tablespoon flaxseed oil

½ lemon, juiced

2 tablespoons raw sesame seeds, unhulled

3 tablespoons Nama Shoyu soy sauce

2 tablespoons water

1 teaspoon kelp or dulse powder

½ clove garlic, peeled and crushed

2 teaspoons ginger powder or 1 teaspoon fresh grated ginger

Blend all the ingredients in a blender until smooth.

Butternut Tahini Dressing

(Makes ½ cup)

⅓ cup butternut squash, peeled, seeded, and shredded in food processor

1 teaspoon raw tahini

1 tablespoon cold-pressed olive or 1 tablespoon raw apple cider vinegar

1 teaspoon nutiritional yeast

1 tablespoon tamari to taste

1 teaspoon turmeric powder—optional

Dash of sesame oil

Pinch of sea salt

About 2 tablespoons water or nut milk

Blend all ingredients in a blender until smooth.

Cucumber Dressing/Dip

1 cucumber

½ avocado

½ cup cashews, soaked for several hours

1 teaspoon olive oil

1 tablespoon dill, preferably fresh

½ teaspoon Herbamare seasoning salt or sea salt with some dried herbs such as oregano, sage, and thyme sprinkled in

Blend all ingredients in a food processor or blender until smooth.

Pear-Mint Dressing

1 pear

¼ cup fresh mint

2 teaspoons apple cider vinegar

Pinch of sea salt

2 tablespoons soaked cashews

2 tablespoons olive oil

Water as needed to blend

Blend all ingredients in a blender until smooth.

* *

Meyer Lemon Dressing

(Makes ½ cup)

2 whole Meyer lemons, peeled but with white pith intact

1 tablespoon raw honey

½ cup extra-virgin olive oil

Pinch of sea salt

Freshly ground black pepper to taste

Blend lemons and honey on high speed in a blender for one minute to break up the seeds and pith. While blender is running, slowly pour in the olive oil. Season with sea salt and pepper to taste.

* *

Sweet Miso Dressing

(Makes 1 cup)

¼ cup unpasteurized white miso

2–3 tablespoons raw agave nectar

¼ cup mirin

2 tablespoons sesame oil

2 tablespoons lemon juice

2 tablespoons chopped ginger

Blend all ingredients in a blender until smooth. Keeps in the refrigerator for three to four days.

* *

Mac-Lime Dressing

¼ cup macadamia oil or grapeseed oil

1 tablespoon lime juice

1 tablespoon grapefruit juice (preferably pink grapefruit)

Coarse sea salt to taste

Freshly ground black pepper to taste

1 teaspoon crushed coriander seeds or a dash of cumin—optional

Whisk all the ingredients together in a bowl or blend in a blender until combined.

* *

Lemon-Lime-Mac Dressing

Juice from 1–2 lemons

Juice from 1–2 limes

⅓ cup macadamia oil

Coarse sea salt to taste

Whisk all ingredients together in a bowl or blend in a blender until well integrated.

* *

Mango Sauce/Dressing

1 ripe mango, peeled and pitted

1 small red chili pepper

3–4 tablespoons coconut water or lime juice

Coarse sea salt to taste

Blend the flesh of the mango with the red chili pepper and enough coconut water or lime juice to achieve the desired consistency. You may transfer this sauce to a squeeze bottle and use it to drizzle over salad or sliced fruit.

* *

Lemon Vinaigrette

3 tablespoons extra-virgin olive oil

1 tablespoon lemon juice

Coarse sea salt and freshly ground black pepper to taste

Whisk all ingredients together until well combined.

* *

Creamy Citrus Dressing

(Makes 1 cup)

½ small avocado, peeled and pitted

½ cup orange juice

3 tablespoons lime juice

¼ cup cilantro, chopped

½ green onion, coarsely chopped

1 teaspoon shallot, chopped

¼ small jalepeno pepper

¼ teaspoon sea salt

¼ cup extra-virgin olive oil

Freshly ground black pepper to taste

Place all ingredients except the olive oil in a blender and blend on high until smooth. With the blender running, slowly add the olive oil and allow it to emulsify until it reaches a rich, creamy consistency.

Spicy Almond Dressing

(Makes 2 cups)

1 cup almond butter

2 Roma tomatoes

¼ cup Nama Shoyu soy sauce

2 teaspoons lime juice

1 tablespoon maple syrup, raw honey, or raw agave nectar

½ teaspoon miso

2 inch fresh ginger

½-inch piece lemongrass

3–4 Thai chili peppers

½ teaspoon sea salt

Blend all ingredients in a food processor or blender until completely smooth. Thin with water as needed.

Ginger Miso Dressing

(Makes 2 cups)

3 tablespoons white miso

3 tablespoons raw agave nectar

2 tablespoons apple cider vinegar

3 tablespoons sesame oil

2 tablespoons lemon juice

3 tablespoons chopped ginger

Blend all ingredients in a food processor or blender until completely smooth.

Creamy Sesame Dressing

(Makes 1 cup)

¼ cup Nama Shoyu soy sauce

¼ cup tahini

2 tablespoons sesame oil

1 tablespoon raw agave syrup

2 tablespoons apple cider vinegar

½ teaspoon sea salt

½ inch fresh ginger

2 tablespoons olive oil

½ teaspoon lime juice

Blend all ingredients in a food processor or blender until smooth.

Creamy Thai Dressing

¼ cup sesame oil

3 tablespoons Nama Shoyu soy sauce

2 tablespoons olive oil

2 tablespoons lime juice

2 teaspoons maple syrup or raw agave nectar

1 tablespoon red chili flakes

½ teaspoon sea salt

2 tablespoons chopped raw cashews

Blend all ingredients in a blender until smooth.

Potato Salad Dressing

1 tablespoon tahini

Pinch of ground cumin

1 tablespoon lemon juice

1 tablespoon water

1 tablespoon fresh parsley

Dash of Nama Shoyu soy sauce

Dash of agave syrup

Pinch of sea salt

Pinch of chili powder

Blend all ingredients in a food processor or blender until smooth. Dressing will be thick and will thin out when added to raw vegetables.

Use this with diced raw jicama, raw turnips, or other raw vegetables for a raw "potato salad."

Lemon Tahini Dressing/Dip

¼ cup soaked flax seeds

2 green onions

¼ bell pepper

1 stalk celery

Juice of 1 lemon

1 cup of raw tahini

Nama Shoyu soy sauce, tamari, or Bragg's liquid aminos to taste

Water as needed to achieve desired consistency.

Juice the lemon and add lemon juice to blender along with pepper, onion, celery, and flax seeds. Blend until smooth. Add one-quarter of the tahini at a time, blending until smooth. Add Bragg's or tamari to taste. Add water as necessary.

Green Dressing Dip

¼ cup soaked almonds

½ bunch cilantro

3 tablespoons fresh parsley, chopped

1 clove garlic

1 tablespoon lemon juice

2 tablespoons olive oil

1 tablespoon Nama Shoyu soy sauce, tamari, or Bragg's liquid aminos

2–3 tablespoons water as needed

½ teaspoon of raw honey

1 teaspoon cumin

Dash of cayenne

Blend all ingredients together in a blender until smooth.

Lavender Dressing

3 tablespoons olive oil

1 tablespoons apple cider vinegar

½ tablespoon lemon juice

1 tablespoon raw honey

½ teaspoon Dijon mustard

½ teaspoon dried lavender flowers, ground or whole

Blend all ingredients in a blender until smooth.

Avocado-Cashew-Tarragon Dressing

½ cup cashews

¼ cup water

2 tablespoons fresh tarragon

½ clove garlic

1 tablespoon apple cider vinegar

1 teaspoon lemon juice

3 tablespoons olive oil

Water as needed to blend

Blend all ingredients in a blender until smooth. Pour over salad when ready to serve.

Raw Hummus

1 cup chick pea sprouts, sprouted overnight (see Day Sixteen about sprouting)

Juice of 1 lemon or lime

2 tablespoons fresh orange juice

1 clove garlic

2 tablespoons raw tahini

Pinch of ground cumin and/or paprika to taste

Blend all ingredients in a blender until smooth.

Raw Mayonnaise

½ cup soaked almonds or cashews

½ cup water (to desired consistency)

2 tablespoons lemon juice

½ clove garlic

½ tablespoon raw honey—optional

¼ teaspoon sea salt (or dried seaweed)

Raw apple cider vinegar to taste

Extra-virgin olive oil to taste

Blend all the ingredients except the olive oil in a blender until smooth. With the blender still running, gradually add olive oil and blend until emulsified.

* *

"Alfredo" Sauce

1 cup raw cashews, soaked overnight and rinsed

½ teaspoon onion powder

¼ teaspoon garlic powder

Sea salt to taste

Water as needed to achieve desired consistency

Place all ingredients except the water and salt in a blender and pulse a few times until powdery. Add water gradually until you reach the desired consistency. Add sea salt to taste.

* *

SOUPS

* *

Cream of Cauliflower Soup

(Makes 1 to 2 servings)

1 cup cauliflower

1 cup water

¼ cup raw cashews or pine nuts

1 tablespoon lemon juice

Sea salt to taste

Blend all ingredients in a blender until thick and smooth.

* *

Honeydew-Cucumber Soup

(Makes 2 servings)

½ honeydew melon, peeled and chopped

½ cucumber, peeled, seeded, and sliced

Several sprigs of mint, stems removed

Blend the cucumber and mint in a blender, add the melon, and blend on low speed. Chill and serve.

Green Spinach Soup

(Makes 2 servings)

1 avocado

1 red bell pepper

3 tablespoons fresh cilantro

1 cup spinach

1 lemon, seeded

1 cup water

½ small jalapeno pepper

¼ teaspoon sea salt—optional

Blend all ingredients in a blender until creamy. Garnish with thinly sliced napa cabbage, red cabbage, or dulse leaves or flakes.

Mediterranean Soup

(Makes 1 quart)

1 cup spinach

1 stalk celery

1 teaspoon oregano

1 teaspoon thyme

½ red bell pepper

½ avocado

½ cucumber

½ jalapeno pepper

2 tablespoons lime juice

¾ cup water

Dulse leaves or flakes—optional

Blend all ingredients in a blender until smooth.

• •

Lemon-Mint Soup

2 apples

½ lemon

2 cups mesclun or spring salad mix

2 tablespoons Bragg's liquid aminos

1 avocado

1 cup fresh mint

4 cups water

Blend ingredients together in a blender until creamy.

• •

Raw Orange-Tomato Soup

3 tomatoes, diced

2 oranges, peeled and sliced

¼ cup sun-dried tomato slices, soaked for thirty minutes and drained

1 inch fresh ginger, peeled

Fresh basil leaves for garnish

Process all ingredients in a blender or food processor. Garnish with fresh basil leaf, and serve with a side of fresh sprouts.

• •

Raw Vegetable Delight Soup

(Makes 2 servings)

1 cup tomatoes, chopped

1 clove garlic, minced

2 cups onion, chopped

1 cucumber, peeled and diced

1 yellow squash, chopped

1 zucchini, chopped

1 cup celery, diced

2 cups red bell pepper, diced

½ ear corn, kernels cut off cob

2 teaspoons sea salt

2 teaspoons dried dill or ½ teaspoon fresh dill

Blend all ingredients in a blender or food processor to desired consistency. Garnish with slices of cucumber and a sprinkle of fresh dill.

Celeriac and Green Apple Soup

(Makes 2 cups)

2 cups celeriac (celery root), peeled, chopped

½ cup chopped green apple plus ½ cup diced fine for garnish

1 cup raw macadamia nuts, soaked for one hour or more

1 cup water

1 tablespoon coconut butter

3 tablespoons extra-virgin olive oil

2 tablespoons fresh lemon juice

2 tablespoons minced chives

Fresh, chopped parsley, thyme, or rosemary for garnish

Blend celeriac and green apple in a blender until smooth. Pass mixture through a sieve or strainer, and discard pulp. Pour the strained liquid back into the blender along with the macadamia nuts, water, coconut butter, olive oil, and lemon juice. Blend thoroughly. Strain once again if desired. Season with sea salt and freshly ground pepper to taste.

Thai Soup

(Makes 1 serving)

1 cucumber

½ large avocado

1 lime, juiced

2 cloves garlic

3 leaves curly kale

¼ teaspoon turmeric powder

¼ inch fresh ginger

1 cup water

Blend all ingredients together in a blender to desired consistency.

Energy Soup

(Makes 2 servings)

2 medium beets, trimmed

2 medium carrots, trimmed

½ cucumber, peeled

½ cup mashed avocado

⅓ cup cilantro leaves, loosely packed

3 cups water

2 tablespoons rice vinegar

1 tablespoon Nama Shoyu soy sauce or tamari

1 clove garlic, peeled and crushed

1 small chili pepper, stemmed and seeded

½ teaspoon cumin

1 cup corn, freshly cut off cob

Grate the carrots, beets, and cucumber, and stir together in a bowl. Blend 3 cups of this grated mixture in a blender until smooth. Combine the blended mixture with the grated vegetables and the corn. Stir well and serve.

Raw Corn Chowder

2 ears fresh corn, kernels removed

3 medium tomatoes, chopped

1 red bell pepper, chopped

1 cucumber

½ cup rough-cut okra

Handful of fresh basil leaves

Juice of ½ lemon

Small handful of dulse—optional

½ avocado

Process cucumber, tomato, okra, basil, dulse, and lemon juice in a food processor, and pulse until blended but still chunky. Add bell pepper, corn, and avocado, and blend to desired consistency. I prefer it with some texture and chunkiness to it.

Creamy Carrot-Ginger Soup

(Makes 2 servings)

1½ cups fresh carrot juice

½ small, ripe avocado

⅓ cup coconut meat from a fresh, young coconut

1 tablespoon lime juice

2 teaspoons minced ginger

Pinch of cayenne pepper

Pinch of sea salt

A few sprigs of cilantro for garnish

Blend all ingredients together in a blender until smooth. Garnish with cilantro leaves.

Broccoli Soup

(Makes 3 servings)

2 tablespoons raw sunflower seeds, soaked for at least thirty minutes and rinsed

3 shitake mushrooms, fresh or dried

2 teaspoons Nama Shoyu soy sauce

½ head celery

1 inch fresh ginger

1 cucumber

1 lemon, peel removed

1½ cups broccoli tops

1 tomato

1 clove garlic, peeled

2 tablespoons extra-virgin olive oil

2 tablespoons raw tahini

¼ cup red onion, diced

Pinch of cayenne pepper to taste

½ cup water

Sprig of fresh cilantro

If using dried shitake mushrooms, combine the 2 teaspoons Nama Shoyu soy sauce with ¼ cup of water and soak for at least one hour. If using fresh mushrooms, marinate them in the 2 teaspoons of soy sauce for one hour.

Remove the mushrooms from the marinade, and set aside. Juice celery, ginger, cucumber, and lemon in a juicer. Add the juice to the remaining ingredients, including the soy sauce marinade. Blend all ingredients in a blender until smooth. Garnish with the marinated mushrooms and a few cilantro leaves.

* *

Pepper Soup

(Makes 2 servings)

1 yellow bell pepper, cored and chopped

1 red bell pepper, cored and chopped

1 green bell pepper, cored and chopped

1 large tomato, diced

½ cup parsley or cliantro (or a blend of both), chopped

½ cup basil leaves, loosely packed

¼ cup onion, chopped

½ apple, cored and chopped

½ cup raw sesame seeds, freshly ground in a coffee grinder or food processor

2 tablespoons unpasteurized miso

3 tablespoons raw apple cider vinegar

¼ cup Bragg's liquid aminos or Nama Shoyu soy sauce

½ habanero pepper

½ teaspoon salt

Freshly ground black pepper to taste

2 cups water

Blend all ingredients together in a blender until smooth.

* *

Papaya-Mint Bisque

(Makes 2 servings)

2 tablespoons fresh mint leaves, torn

1 large or 2 small Hawaiian papayas, chilled and seeded

¼–⅓ cup water

1 lime, juiced

1 tablespoon fresh pineapple or fresh orange juice

Puree all ingredients in a food processor until smooth. Garnish with mint leaves and halved red grapes.

* *

Raw Borscht

(Makes 3 to 4 servings)

1 cup water
1 beet, peeled
1 inch fresh ginger, peeled
2 cloves garlic, peeled
3 bay leaves
Blend all ingredients together in a blender and set aside.
1 cup of water
1 carrot
1 stalk celery
1 tablespoon apple cider vinegar
2 teaspoons of raw honey or raw agave nectar
¼ cup extra-virgin olive oil
Sea salt to taste
Blend these ingredients together in a blender for thirty seconds
¼ head cabbage, grated
1 carrot, grated
½ bunch parsley
Add grated ingredients to blended mixtures and serve.

Cucumber-Dill Soup

(Makes 2 servings)

1 cucumber
½ cup fresh dill
1 small avocado
2 leaves dinosaur kale, stems removed
1 stalk celery
2 tablespoons lime juice
1 clove garlic
Blend all ingredients together in a blender or food processor to desired consistency.

Gazpacho

(Makes 2 servings)

1 leaf kale, finely chopped

3 tablespoons fresh basil, chopped

3 tablespoons fresh cilantro, chopped

1 tomato, diced

½ stalk celery, diced

½ red bell pepper, diced

½ avocado

2 tablespoons lime juice

2 tablespoons extra-virgin olive oil

⅓ cup water

Pulse all ingredients in a food processor until combined but still chunky. Allow to sit for thirty minutes or longer before serving.

Butternut-Leek Soup

(Makes 3 to 4 servings)

1 small, fresh leek

1 bunch celery

½ butternut squash, peeled and deseeded

1 small avocado

2 tablespoons raw tahini

4 tablespoons flaxseed oil or olive oil

1 teaspoon sea salt

3 tablespoons chives, minced

Freshly ground black pepper to taste

Juice the leeks and the celery in a juicer. Shred the squash in a food processor. Blend the celery-leek juice in a blender with the shredded squash. Add water to reach desired consistency. Garnish with minced chives.

Pumpkin Pie in a Bowl Soup

(Makes 2 cups)

2 cups fresh carrot juice

½ cup raw sweet potato, peeled and cubed

Stevia to taste

¼ avocado

¼ teaspoon pumpkin pie spice or ⅛ teaspoon cinnamon combined with a pinch of ground cloves and a pinch of nutmeg

Place all ingredients in a blender, and blend until smooth. May be stored in an airtight container in the refrigerator for up to thirty-six hours.

SALADS

Lettuce and Persimmon Salad with Walnut Butter Dressing

1 head romaine lettuce, chopped

2 large Fuyu persimmons, chopped

½ large fennel bulb, sliced thinly

2 large handfuls of alfalfa sprouts

1 tablespoon hemp seeds—optional

Place all ingredients in a large bowl, and toss with walnut dressing.

For the Walnut Dressing:

1 tablespoon walnut butter or any other raw nut butter of your choice

Juice from 1 large orange

Blend in a blender until smooth, or place in a jar and shake vigorously until combined.

Creamy Asian Salad

(Makes 2 to 4 servings)

For the Salad:

1 cup mung bean sprouts

1 cup shredded green or purple cabbage

½ red bell pepper, thinly sliced

½ cup sugar snap peas

¼ cup mushrooms (shitake or button), sliced

2 tablespoons fresh cilantro, chopped

1 tablespoon fresh basil, chopped

½ clove garlic, chopped

Mix all ingredients together, and set aside.

For the Dressing:

½ inch fresh ginger, chopped

½ cup cold-pressed olive oil

1 teaspoon sesame oil

1 clove garlic

2 tablespoons lemon juice

3 whole dates, pitted

1 tablespoon Nama Shoyu soy sauce

2 tablespoons water

Blend all ingredients together in a blender until smooth. One hour before serving, pour half the dressing over the salad. Mix thoroughly.

Shaved Asparagus Salad with Mustard Seed

(Makes 2 servings)

½ bunch asparagus, tips cut off and bracts shaved with vegetable peeler

5 radishes, sliced thin

⅓ cup fresh orange juice

2 tablespoons apple cider vinegar

½ teaspoon mustard seed

¼ cup extra-virgin olive oil

Sea salt and freshly ground black pepper to taste

1 tablespoon orange zest

Wash asparagus and trim ends.

For the Mustard Seed Vinaigrette:

Blend vinegar, olive oil, mustard seeds, and orange juice in a blender until smooth.

Toss shaved asparagus, sliced radishes, coarse pepper, sea salt, and vinaigrette. Garnish with asparagus tips and orange zest.

Green Salad with Cucumbers and Mangoes

2–3 hearts or ½ large head romaine lettuce, torn into bite-sized pieces

2–3 baby cucumbers or ½ large cucumber, sliced

2–3 mangoes, cubed

3–4 medium tomatoes, diced

½ cup cilantro, chopped

Combine all ingredients, toss, and serve.

Classic Chopped Salad

(Makes 2 servings)

½ cup fresh green beans

2 ears fresh corn, kernels cut from cob

½ yellow bell pepper, chopped

1 large carrot, chopped

1 cup grape tomatoes, sliced in half

½ zucchini, chopped

1 tablespoon fresh chives, minced

2 tablespoons fresh lemon juice

½ teaspoon fresh garlic, diced

Blend all ingredients together in a blender until smooth.

Raw Corn Salad

(Makes 2 to 3 servings)

4 ears fresh corn, kernels cut from cobs

4 stalks celery, chopped

1 red bell pepper, chopped

4–5 radishes, chopped

1 medium avocado, chopped

Juice of 1 lime

½ head romaine lettuce

1 cup arugula

Arrange romaine lettuce and arugula on two or three plates. Mix the other ingredients thoroughly, spoon into a tea cup or small bowl, and turn onto the lettuce.

Refreshing Summer Salad

(Makes 1 to 2 servings)

1 cup fresh arugula or spinach

1 avocado, sliced

1 bulb fennel, julienned

½ cup sweet cherry or grape tomatoes, halved

1 orange bell pepper, julienned

¼ cup sliced scallions

1 tablespoon fresh dill—optional

¼ cup fresh lemon juice

Liquid stevia, several drops to taste

Combine all the vegetables, and toss together.

Fennel Salad

1 large fennel bulb, shredded

1 red bell pepper, cut into two-inch-long thin strips

1 cucumber, diced

½ avocado, chopped

Juice of 1 lemon or lime

2 tablespoons hemp seeds

Toss all ingredients together in a bowl, and enjoy.

Summer Green Salad with Avocado and Cashew Tarragon Dressing

(Makes 2 to 4 servings)

3 cups greens, such as watercress, chard, and arugula

2 cups spinach

1 tablespoon fresh mint

½ cup baby tomatoes, cut into quarters

½ cucumber, diced

1 red pepper, sliced or diced

1 avocado, cut into a fan

1 tablespoon lemon juice

2 teaspoons olive oil

Combine greens, spinach, red pepper, and cucumber. Just before serving, toss the salad with the lemon juice and olive oil. Top with avocado.

For the Dressing:

½ cup cashews, soaked overnight

¼ cup water

2 tablespoons fresh tarragon

½ clove garlic

1 tablespoon apple cider vinegar

1 teaspoon lemon juice

3 tablespoons olive oil

Water as needed to blend

Blend all ingredients together in a blender until smooth. Pour over salad when ready to serve.

Avocado-Kale Salad

½ head kale

1 avocado

4-5 radishes, sliced

1 cucumber, sliced

¼ cup raw almonds

2 tablespoons lemon juice

Sea salt to taste

Nutritional yeast—optional

Combine kale and avocado. Add cucumber, radishes, and almonds, and toss gently. Add lemon juice, sea salt, and other spices. Toss and serve.

Asian Coleslaw

½ large napa cabbage, shredded

½ medium daikon radish, grated

1 cucumber, grated

½ bunch cilantro, chopped

⅓ cup wakame flakes, soaked for twenty to thirty minutes

1 avocado

Juice of 1 large lime

Mix all ingredients together and serve.

Mock Tuna Salad Using Juicer Pulp

Carrot or vegetable pulp

Raw mayonnaise

Celery, diced

Onions, chopped

Spices to taste

Add raw mayonnaise (see recipe below) to your juicer pulp. Add other veggies to taste (scallions, celery, etc.). Add spices to taste.

For the Raw Mayonnaise:

½ cup soaked almonds or cashews

½ cup water (to desired consistency)

2 tablespoons lemon juice

½ clove garlic

½ tablespoon raw honey—optional

¼ teaspoon sea salt (or dried seaweed)

Raw apple cider vinegar to taste

Extra-virgin olive oil to taste

Blend all the ingredients except the olive oil in a blender until smooth. With the blender still running, gradually add olive oil and blend until emulsified. Lasts in the refrigerator for up to one week.

Avocado and Apple Salad with Wakame

(Makes 2 servings)

2 teaspoons extra-virgin olive oil

½ teaspoon lemon juice

Sea salt and pepper to taste

½ avocado, thinly sliced

½ apple, peeled, cored, and julienned

2 teaspoons wakame, soaked for twenty to thirty minutes and then drained and julienned

Whisk together the olive oil and lemon juice. Season with salt and pepper. Add the avocado, apple, and wakame. Toss gently.

Carrot-Raisin Salad

4 large carrots, grated

½ cup raisins

Juice of ½ lemon

Soak the raisins in water for at least one-half hour. Combine grated carrots. Add the soaked raisins and lemon juice, and mix together before serving.

"Pizza" Salad

(Makes 2 servings)

6–8 unsulfured sun-dried tomatoes, soaked in lukewarm water until soft, chopped

¼–½ pound fresh baby greens

¼ cup fresh basil, chopped

1 tablespoon fresh oregano, chopped

1 tablespoon lemon juice

1 clove garlic, minced—optional

1 teaspoon raw honey or raw agave nectar—optional

Sea salt and freshly ground black pepper to taste

Combine all the ingredients, and toss well.

* *

Thai Cucumber Salad

1 cucumber, chopped

2 Roma tomatoes, diced

½ avocado, chopped

½ cup sun-dried tomatoes, soaked four hours, drained, and diced

2 mint leaves, minced

2 basil leaves, minced

½ teaspoon finely diced fresh ginger

Juice of 1 lime

2 tablespoons hemp seeds

Toss all ingredients together in a bowl, and enjoy.

* *

Spinach Salad with Cashews, Avocado, and Cranberries

1 cup baby spinach

⅓ cup raw cashews

¼ cup dried cranberries

½ avocado, organic

1 teaspoon lime juice

Cut avocado into bite-sized chunks, and sprinkle with lime juice. Toss all ingredients together.

* *

Lavender-Berry Salad

1 cup baby greens

1 tomato, sliced

2 ripe peaches, sliced

½ cup strawberries, sliced

½ cup blueberries

½ cup microgreens

Combine all ingredients, and toss gently.

For the Lavender Dressing:

6 tablespoons olive oil

2 tablespoons apple cider vinegar

1 tablespoon lemon juice

2 tablespoons raw honey

1 teaspoon Dijon mustard

1 teaspoon dried lavender flowers, ground or whole

Whisk all the ingredients together, and allow to sit for about thirty minutes. Pour over the salad, toss, and serve.

* *

Ginger-Carrot Coleslaw

(Makes 2 servings)

2 carrots, grated

1 cup red cabbage, shredded

½ cup raisins

2 tablespoons sunflower seeds

2 teaspoons pumpkin seeds

Toss all ingredients together until combined.

For the Dressing:

1 teaspoon raw honey

1 tablespoon lemon juice

2 teaspoons grated ginger

2 tablespoons cold-pressed oil of your choice

Dash of sea salt

Dissolve the honey in the lemon juice. Add the remaining ingredients. Pour over the salad, and toss. Allow salad to marinate for about fifteen to thirty minutes.

* *

Cinnamon Spice Salad

(Makes 2 servings)

½ pound romaine or baby lettuce, chopped

1 cup cherry or grape tomatoes, sliced in half

1 teaspoon cinnamon

1 teaspoon ground cloves

1 clove garlic, chopped

1 teaspoon fresh oregano, chopped

1 teaspoon fresh thyme, chopped

2 tablespoons fresh lemon juice

Raw honey or raw agave nectar to taste

4 raw olives, chopped

Sea salt and freshly ground black pepper to taste

Combine all the ingredients, and toss well.

* *

Guacamole Salad

(Makes 2 to 4 servings)

2 Haas avocados, finely chopped

4 ripe Holland tomatoes, diced, or 2 cups grape tomatoes, sliced in half

1 bunch cilantro, chopped

1 pound baby romaine, mesclun, or regular romaine lettuce, chopped

Juice of 1 lime

Several drops of liquid stevia or 1 teaspoon of raw honey or raw agave nectar—optional

Celtic sea salt and freshly ground black pepper to taste

Dash of cayenne—optional

Combine all the ingredients, and toss well.

* *

Seaweed Salad

½ cup dried hijiki seaweed, soaked in water for ten to twenty minutes or until softened, rinsed, drained, and chopped

1 apple, diced

1 cup cucumber, sliced thinly into quarter moons

½ cup grated carrots

1 teaspoon freshly grated ginger, or to taste

2 tablespoons sesame oil to taste

1 tablespoon apple cider vinegar

1 tablespoon soy sauce or tamari

1 clove garlic, minced

2 tablespoons sesame seeds

Combine all ingredients, and toss well.

* *

Arame Seaweed Salad

½ cup dried arame seaweed, soaked in water for ten to twenty minutes or until softened, rinsed, drained, and chopped

1 cup plum tomatoes, diced

½ cup celery, thinly sliced

¼ cup fresh cilantro, finely chopped

2 tablespoons rice vinegar, or to taste

Drizzle of tamari or soy sauce

1 tablespoon sliced almonds

Combine all ingredients, and toss well.

* *

Seaweed Salad

½ cup dried hijiki seaweed, soaked in water for ten to twenty minutes or until softened, rinsed, drained, and chopped

1 apple, diced

1 cup cucumber, sliced thinly into quarter moons

½ cup grated carrots

1 teaspoon freshly grated ginger, or to taste

2 tablespoons sesame oil to taste

1 tablespoon apple cider vinegar

1 tablespoon soy sauce or tamari

1 clove garlic, minced

2 tablespoons sesame seeds

Combine all ingredients, and toss well.

* *

Wakame Seaweed Salad

½ cup dried wakame seaweed, soaked in water for five to ten minutes or until softened, rinsed, drained, and chopped

1 cup cabbage, shredded

½ cup carrots, shredded

½ cup mushrooms, chopped

1 clove garlic, finely minced

1 tablespoon apple cider vinegar

1 tablespoon tamari or soy sauce

1 tablespoon sesame oil

In a bowl, combine the ingredients, and adjust the oil to taste, if needed.

* *

ENTREES

. . . .

Zucchini Pasta

1 small to medium zucchini per person (you also may substitute rutabaga or turnip)

Run the zucchini or other vegetable through a Saladacco shredder or food processor for long "spaghetti" or simply cut by hand into thin shreds.

Rinse and allow to drain in a colander for a few minutes. Top with Italian Tomato Sauce or Pesto Sauce (see recipes below).

For the Italian Tomato Sauce:

3 large fresh vine-ripened organic tomatoes, ⅓ chopped into chunks, ⅔ pureed in a blender or food processor

1 clove garlic, peeled and crushed

¼ cup fresh basil and oregano, mixed

1 tablespoon dried Italian herb mixture (including basil, oregano, thyme, and parsley)

Freshly ground black pepper to taste

¼ onion, minced

¼ cup extra-virgin olive oil

2 tablespoons raw apple cider vinegar

1 tablespoon raw honey or raw agave nectar

Dash of cinnamon

Blend all ingredients in a blender until smooth. Serve over Zucchini Pasta.

For the Pesto Sauce:

½ bunch fresh basil

½ cup pine nuts or walnuts, or combine both

1 clove garlic, peeled and crushed

½ cup extra-virgin olive oil

Fresh black pepper to taste

Chop the basil together with the nuts for a few seconds in a food processor. Add all the remaining ingredients, and pulse into a thick and chunky paste. Serve tossed with Zucchini Pasta.

. . . .

Raw Sushi

(Makes 8 rolls)

2 sheets nori seaweed

2 romaine leaves

½ cup alfalfa sprouts

½ cucumber, julienned

½ carrot, shredded or julienned

½ avocado, sliced—optional

Place the nori sheet in front of you. Lay one leaf of romaine lettuce horizontally on the top of the nori sheet on the side closest to you. Lay the sprouts, cucumber pieces, and carrot pieces horizontally following the line of the romaine leaf. Carefully roll it tightly. Moisten the end of the nori farthest from you with water, and seal it like an envelope. Slice the roll with a sharp knife down the middle or cut into smaller one- to two-inch pieces.

For the Japanese "Rice":

(Makes about 1 cup)

½ cup chopped parsnips

¼ cup raw pine nuts

1 tablespoon raw honey

⅓ tablespoon rice vinegar

1 tablespoon raw Teriyaki Sauce (see below)

Pulse the parsnips, pine nuts, honey, and vinegar in a food processor until the mixture resembles brown rice. Add the sauce, and mix well. Serve alongside Raw Sushi (see above).

For the Teriyaki Sauce:

¼ cup Nama Shoyu soy sauce

¼ cup raw agave nectar

¼ teaspoon ginger, whole

½ teaspoon minced garlic

Drizzle of sesame oil

Blend all the ingredients together in a blender, and use as a dipping sauce.

* *

Endive Bruschetta

(Makes about 5 servings)

1 Roma tomato, diced

½ clove garlic, minced

¼ cup packed fresh basil

Sea salt and freshly ground black pepper to taste

½ head endive, separated into leaves

Combine the tomato, garlic, basil, salt, and pepper. Place a heaping tablespoon of the mixture on each endive leaf.

* *

Indian Curry Vegetables

(Makes 2 to 3 servings)

4 apricots, sliced (or 2–3 dates, pits removed), soaked for twenty to thirty minutes

¼ cup warm water

3 cups assorted chopped vegetables such as cauliflower, broccoli, zucchini, carrots, green beans, red bell peppers, collard greens, or spinach

2 tablespoons minced spring onion, red onion, or other onion

1 tablespoon minced ginger

1 clove garlic

¼ teaspoon curry powder

¼ teaspoon coriander

¼ teaspoon sea salt

½ tablespoon Nama Shoyu soy sauce

2 tablespoons cilantro, minced

Soak apricots or dates in ¼ cup warm water for twenty minutes. Toss all the vegetables together. Place the remaining ingredients, except the cilantro, in a blender or food processor along with the apricots (or dates) and the soaking water. Process on high speed for thirty seconds or as long as it takes to blend the apricots (or dates) into a thick paste. Toss the vegetables together with the spiced sauce. Allow the vegetables to marinate for several hours before serving.

* *

• •

Raw Ravioli

(Makes 16 raviolis)

1 large turnip, peeled

1 tablespoon extra-virgin olive oil

½ cup pine nuts, soaked for at least two hours

1 cup macadamia nuts, soaked for at least two hours

2 teaspoons fresh rosemary, minced

2 teaspoons fresh parsley, minced

2 teaspoons fresh thyme, minced

1 tablespoon nutritional yeast

½ teaspoon salt

½ teaspoon freshly ground black pepper

2 teaspoons apple cider vinegar

¼ cup water as needed

Using a vegetable peeler, a mandoline, or a sharp knife, cut turnips into sixteen very thin slices. Coat turnip slices in olive oil, and allow to marinate for at least one hour.

Rinse pine nuts and macadamia nuts, and drain well for at least ten minutes. Place in a food processor fitted with the S-shaped blade, and process on high speed for ten seconds. Add rosemary, parsley, thyme, nutritional yeast, sea salt, black pepper, and apple cider vinegar. Blend on high speed for about twenty seconds while adding water through the top until you reach a smooth, cheesy consistency. Scoop 1 tablespoon of this mixture onto each turnip slice, and fold the slice in half. Cover with Sun-Dried Tomato-Sage Sauce (see recipe below).

For the Sun-Dried Tomato-Sage Sauce:

(Makes 1 cup)

2–3 tablespoons sun-dried tomatoes, chopped and soaked in ½ cup water

½ cup filtered water

1 cup Roma tomatoes, chopped

1 tablespoon beets, shredded

1 tablespoon extra-virgin olive oil

2 teaspoons fresh basil, minced

2 teaspoons fresh parsley, minced

½ teaspoon Nama Shoyu soy sauce

½ teaspoon nutritional yeast

¼ teaspoon fresh oregano, minced

¼ teaspoon fresh thyme, minced

¼ teaspoon sea salt

Pinch of freshly ground black pepper

1 teaspoon rubbed sage

Raw agave nectar to taste

Soak sun-dried tomatoes in ½ cup of water for at least thirty minutes. Drain and reserve liquid. Blend sun-dried tomatoes, Roma tomatoes, soak water, beets, olive oil, basil, parsley, Nama Shoyu, nutritional yeast, oregano, thyme, salt, pepper, and sage in a blender to desired consistency.

Sea Vegetable Wraps

½ head romaine lettuce

½ carrot, shredded

¼ cup fresh alfalfa or broccoli sprouts

2 sheets of nori, cut into one- by three-inch strips

Place a spoonful of sauce (see recipe below) at the top of a lettuce leaf. Add a pinch of sprouts, shredded carrot, and a strip of nori. Fold the top of the leaf over, and roll the entire lettuce leaf up tightly.

For the Sauce:

2 tablespoons dulse flakes

1 tablespoon tahini

1 tablespoon chia seeds, soaked for fifteen minutes

2 tablespoons fresh lemon juice

3 tablespoons water

Blend all ingredients in a blender until smooth. Allow the sauce to sit for fifteen minutes. Add more water if necessary. The sauce should be thick so that it will stay put in the wrap.

Raw Chili

1 zucchini, chopped into ½-inch cubes

1 carrot, chopped into ¼-inch cubes

½ small eggplant, peeled and chopped into ½-inch cubes

1 small Portobello mushroom or 5 shiitake mushrooms, chopped into cubes

3 cloves garlic, crushed

1 medium Roma tomato, chopped into ½-inch cubes

¼ medium red onion, chopped

3½ teaspoons sea salt

1 tablespoon lemon juice

2 tablespoons extra-virgin olive oil

Mix all ingredients together, and place in a quart-sized jar. Press down firmly so that the vegetables are completely immersed in the salt, lemon juice, and oil. Cover and let marinate for at least four to six hours or overnight.

For the Chili Sauce:

1 large tomato

1 cup sun-dried tomatoes, soaked with enough water to cover

¼ cup olive oil

1½ cups purified water

⅛ teaspoon cayenne

½ tablespoon celery seed

½ tablespoon oregano

½ teaspoon cumin

1½ teaspoons chili powder

Blend ingredients on high speed until smooth. Pour blended mixture over marinated vegetables, or pulse together in a food processor.

* *

Mushroom "Fettucini Alfredo"

(Makes 3 to 5 servings)

5–6 medium zucchinis, peeled

With a vegetable peeler, slice thin strands of the zuchinnis. Set aside.

For the Mushroom Sauce:

¾ cup soaked dried mushrooms or 1 cup fresh mushrooms

¾ cup soaked cashews

¾–1 cup water

1 tablespoon extra-virgin olive oil

1 tablespoon raw agave nectar

2 tablespoons fresh lemon juice

¼ teaspoon dried white pepper

Sea salt to taste

Process all ingredients for the mushroom sauce in a blender or food processor until smooth. Add the sauce to the pasta. Toss well, and let sit for half an hour before serving.

* *

Spicy Raw Rice

1 small head cauliflower

¼ head green cabbage

½ hot pepper

½ bunch cilantro

Handful of chopped dulse

½ medium diakon radish

1 inch fresh ginger

Juice of 1 lemon or lime

2 tablespoons hemp seeds—optional

Process all the ingredients except the hemp seed in several batches in your food processor with the S blade until all the vegetables are the about the size of half a grain of rice. Mix in the hemp seeds, and serve as a main course or a side dish.

* *

Beet Stacks with Parsley Pesto and Sweet Pepper–Fennel Cream

(Makes 2 to 3 servings)

3 medium beets, peeled and sliced very thin on a mandoline or with a sharp knife or vegetable peeler

1 tablespoons extra-virgin olive oil

Sea salt and freshly ground black pepper to taste

Toss the beets with the olive oil, and sprinkle with a bit of salt and pepper until the beets are evenly coated.

For the Parsley Pesto:

2 cloves garlic

1½ cups raw pumpkin seeds, soaked for four to six hours, drained, and rinsed

1 cup parsley leaves, well packed

¾ cup extra-virgin olive oil

¾ teaspoon sea salt

Process the garlic in a food processor until finely chopped. Add the remaining ingredients, and process until well combined.

For the Cream Sauce:

1 sweet bell pepper

½ cup carrots, roughly chopped

¼ cup extra-virgin olive oil

1 clove garlic

½ teaspoon sea salt

¾ teaspoon dried fennel seed

Blend the bell pepper, carrot, olive oil, garlic, and salt in a blender until smooth. Add the fennel seed, and blend lightly until just combined.

For the Assembly:

For each stack, begin with one slice of beet. Top with 2 teaspoons of parsley pesto. Cover with another slice of beet. Top with two more teaspoons of pesto and then a third slice of beet. Place a small spoonful of the sweet pepper sauce on top of the third beet. You may want to build several stacks at a time.

* *

Spicy Thai Vegetable Wraps

¼ cup chopped raw cashews

2 teaspoons sesame oil

¼ teaspoon sea salt

2 tablespoons raw agave nectar

¼ cup lemon juice

1 tablespoon chopped ginger

2 teaspoons chopped red chili pepper, seeds included

1 tablespoon Nama Shoyu soy sauce

1 cup raw almond butter

¼ head savoy cabbage, shredded

3 very large collard green leaves

½ large carrot, cut into matchstick-sized pieces

½ large mango, cut lengthwise into strips about ¼-inch thick

1 cup mung bean sprouts

¼ cup cilantro leaves

¼ cup basil leaves, torn

¼ cup mint leaves, torn or cut if leaves are large

For the Dipping Sauce:

3 tablespoons raw honey or raw agave nectar

1 tablespoon extra-virgin olive oil

Pinch of sea salt

Combine cashews, sesame oil, and sea salt, and set aside. Blend the honey or agave nectar, lemon juice, ginger, red chili, and Nama Shoyu soy sauce in a blender until smooth. Add the almond butter, and blend at low speed to combine. Add water to thin if necessary to get a thick, cake batter–like consistency. Add this mixture to the shredded cabbage, and toss well to combine.

Cut out the center rib of each collard green leaf, and divide the leaf in half. Place one-half leaf on a cutting board with the underside facing up. Arrange a few tablespoons of the cabbage mixture evenly across the bottom third of the leaf, leaving about 1½ inches clear at the bottom. Sprinkle some of the cashews over the cabbage. Lay a few sticks of carrot, a few strips of mango, and a few sprouts on top. Add several leaves each of cilantro, basil, and mint. Fold the bottom of the collard leaf up and over the filling, keeping it tight. Tuck the leaf under the ingredients, and roll forward. Place the roll seam side down on a serving dish. Repeat with remaining collard leaves and ingredients. Serve with the Dipping Sauce.

Stuffed Red Peppers

(Makes 2 to 4 servings)

2 red bell peppers, cut in half with seeds/core removed

For the Filling:

1 cup soaked sunflower seeds

½ pint cherry tomatoes

1 stalk celery

½ teaspoon each of cayenne powder, paprika, basil, oregano, and garlic

½ small onion, chopped

2 tablespoons lemon juice

1 tablespoon olive oil

Sea salt to taste

Process all ingredients in a food processor until thick and smooth.

For the Assembly:

Spoon about 2 tablespoons of the filling into each pepper half, and garnish with a parsley leaf.

• •

Garden Herb Roll-ups

(Makes 2 servings)

For the Wraps:

3 large collard leaves

2 Roma tomatoes, thinly sliced

For the Pumpkin Seed Pâté:

1 clove garlic

¼ cup Brazil nuts

¼ cup lemon juice

1½ cups pumpkin seeds, soaked for four to six hours, drained, and rinsed

¼ cup olive oil

½ teaspoon salt

2 tablespoons parsley

2 tablespoons basil

3 tablespoons dill

Chop the garlic in a food processor. Add the Brazil nuts, and process until they are finely chopped. With the blade running, add the lemon juice until the mixture is creamy. Add the pumpkin seeds, olive oil, and the sea salt, and continue to puree this mixture. Add the parsley, basil, and dill, and pulse to finely chop the herbs.

For the Marinated Veggies:

1 cup baby spinach

¾ cup shredded carrots

2 tablespoons onion, very thinly sliced

1 tablespoon extra-virgin olive oil

1 teaspoon lemon juice

Pinch of sea salt

Freshly ground black pepper to taste

Toss all the ingredients in a large bowl, and mix well to combine all the flavors.

For the Assembly:

Lay a collard green on your cutting board with the darker side on the board. Chop off the stem, and trim off any very thick portions of the remaining center stem. Place 6 tablespoons of the pâté on the collard leaf, and spread out a bit, but leave plenty of room for wrapping up the leaf.

Top with a few slices of tomato. Cover with ½ cup of the marinated veggies.

Roll up like a burrito, folding up the top and bottom first and then rolling in the sides.

Mushroom and Cherry Tomato "Fettucini"

(Makes 2 servings)

1–2 goldbar squash, ends trimmed (or substitute another summer squash or zucchini)

Sea salt to taste

1 cup cherry tomatoes, sliced in half

1–2 tablespoons extra-virgin olive oil

Freshly ground black pepper

1 cup mushrooms (field mushrooms with a dense texture work best)

1 teaspoon balsamic vinegar

1 teaspoon Nama Shoyu soy sauce

1–2 whole stalks fresh rosemary

Small handful fresh oregano or 1 teaspoon dried oregano

1 shallot, minced

Using a vegetable peeler or mandoline, slice the squash into wide, thin, fettucine noodle–like ribbons. Discard the seeds at the center. Toss the sliced squash in a colander with ½ teaspoon sea salt. Allow to sit for at least thirty minutes to permit some of the liquid to drain out.

Toss the cherry tomatoes with 1 tablespoon of the olive oil, and season with salt and pepper. Toss well, and allow to marinate for several hours.

Toss the mushrooms with 1 tablespoon of the olive oil, the balsamic vinegar, and the Nama Shoyu soy sauce. Season with salt and pepper. Add rosemary, oregano, and shallot. Toss well, and allow to marinate for several hours.

Toss the squash noodles with the mushroom mixture and the cherry tomatoes. Season with salt and pepper, and garnish with fresh herbs.

Zucchini and Tomato "Lasagne"

(Makes 3 servings)

1 cup raw pine nuts (pignoli), soaked for at least one hour

1 tablespoon lemon juice

1 tablespoon nutritional yeast

½ teaspoon sea salt

1–2 tablespoons water

Place pine nuts, nutritional yeast, lemon juice, and salt in a food processor, and pulse until combined. Add water gradually, and process until the mixture resembles ricotta cheese.

For the Tomato Sauce:

1 cup sun-dried tomatoes, soaked for at least two hours

½ small to medium tomato, diced

2 tablespoons onion, chopped fine

1 tablespoon lemon juice

2 tablespoons extra-virgin olive oil

2 teaspoons raw agave nectar

1 teaspoon sea salt

Drain soaked sun-dried tomatoes, and add to blender, along with remaining ingredients. Blend all ingredients until smooth.

For the Pesto:

1 cup packed basil leaves

¼ cup raw pistachios

3 tablespoons extra-virgin olive oil

½ teaspoon sea salt

Freshly ground black pepper to taste

Blend in food processor until combined but still chunky.

For the Assembly:

1–2 medium zucchini

1 tablespoon extra-virgin olive oil

2 teaspoons fresh oregano, finely chopped

2 teaspoons fresh thyme, finely chopped

Pinch of sea salt

Pinch of freshly ground black pepper

2 medium tomatoes, cut in half and then sliced

Whole basil leaves for garnish

Cut the zucchini into three-inch lengths. Cut lengthwise into very thin slices using a mandoline or a vegetable peeler. Toss the zucchini slices with the olive oil, oregano, thyme, and salt and pepper.

Line the bottom of a nine- by thirteen-inch backing dish with a layer of zucchini slices, overlapping the slices slightly. Spread about a third of the tomato sauce over the slices, and top with small dollops of the pine nut "ricotta" mixture and the pesto, using about a third of each. Layer on a third of the tomato slices. Add another layer of the zucchini slices, and repeat twice more. You may serve immediately, or cover with plastic wrap and allow to sit at room temperature for several hours. Garnish with basil leaves.

* *

Green Curry Coconut Noodles

(Makes 2 to 4 servings)

For the Vegetables:

2 tablespoons extra-virgin olive oil

2 tablespoons white miso

2 teaspoons raw apple cider vinegar

1 tablespoon chopped ginger

1 teaspoon sesame oil

1 green onion, thinly sliced

½ cup yellow squash, thinly sliced

½ cup zucchini, thinly sliced

½ cup mushrooms, diced small

½ carrot, cut into matchsticks

½ cup sliced snap peas, cut on a diagonal into diamond shapes

½ small stalk celery, cut in half lengthwise and then sliced thinly

In a blender, puree the miso, vinegar, ginger, sesame oil, and half the green onion until smooth. Add the second half of the thinly sliced green onion, and toss the sauce with the vegetables. Allow to marinate for at least three hours.

For the Curry:

2 tablespoons grated lemongrass

½ cup coconut meat

2 tablespoons raw cashews, soaked for at least one hour

1 tablespoon lime juice

2 tablespoons jalepeno, chopped

2 green onions

1 tablespoon chopped ginger

2 tablespoons loosely packed basil

1 teaspoon curry powder

1 teaspoon sea salt

¼ cup coconut water

Place all ingredients except coconut water in a blender, and blend until smooth. Add the coconut water a bit at a time until the mixture is the consistency of a thick sauce.

For the Assembly:

¼ cup chopped almonds

½ teaspoon sesame oil

¼ teaspoon sea salt

1 cup coconut "noodles" (from four coconuts)

1 small handful cilantro, chopped

2 tablespoons mint, chopped or torn

2 tablespoons basil, chopped or torn

1 tablespoon sesame seeds (preferably black)

Toss almonds with sesame oil and sea salt.

Add coconut "noodles" to vegetables, add herbs, and toss to combine. Sprinkle with chopped almonds and sesame seeds. Serve with curry sauce.

Pumpkin-Squash Couscous

(Makes 2 servings)

For the Sauce:

1½ cups red bell pepper, chopped

¼ cup habanero pepper, chopped

2 cups yellow bell pepper, chopped

2 cups tomatoes, seeds removed, chopped

¼ cup raw agave nectar

1 shallot, chopped

½ cup extra-virgin olive oil

Sea salt

Freshly ground black pepper

Toss the pepper, agave nectar, shallot, and ¼ cup olive oil

together in a bowl. Season with salt and pepper. Allow mixture to sit for several hours. Drain off the excess liquid. Place pepper mixture in a blender along with the remaining ¼ cup olive oil. Blend until smooth. Set aside.

For the Pumpkin-Squash Mixture:

1 shallot, minced

2 teaspoons fresh thyme

2 teaspoons ground cumin

½ teaspoon ground cinnamon

¼ cup extra-virgin olive oil

2 tablespoons almond milk

2 cups peeled, seeded, diced pumpkin

2 cups yellow squash, cut into half moons

Sea salt

Freshly ground black pepper

¼ cup fresh parsley, minced

¼ cup fresh cilantro, minced

Combine shallot, thyme, cumin, cinnamon, olive oil, and almond milk. Place pumpkin and squash in two separate bowls. Divide the olive oil mixture between the two bowls, toss well, and season with salt and pepper.

Allow pumpkin and squash to marinate for several hours. Combine with parsley and cilantro.

For the Couscous:

3 cups chopped jicama, one-inch-cubes

¼ cup pine nuts

½ cup dried currants

¼ cup almond oil

Coarse sea salt

Pumpkin seeds for garnish

Place jicama in food processor, and pulse several times until chopped to the size of couscous. Press between two kitchen towels or paper towels to remove excess moisture. The mixture should be dry and fluffy.

Chop pine nuts in a food processor until finely chopped. Add to the couscous along with the currants, almond oil, and salt. Combine the squash and pumpkin with the couscous, garnish with pumpkin seeds, and serve with the pepper sauce.

• •

Summer Rolls with Green Papaya

(Makes 4 to 6 rolls)

For the Filling:

½ cup green papaya or green mango, peeled and julienned

½ cup young coconut meat, julienned

½ large carrot, julienned

2 radishes, finely julienned

2 tablespoons julienned ginger

2 tablespoons Nama Shoyu soy sauce

2 tablespoons mirin—optional

2 tablespoons lime juice

1 tablespoon raw agave nectar

½ tablespoon sesame oil

½ long red chili pepper, seeded and minced

Sea salt

Freshly ground black pepper

Combine green papaya (or mango), coconut meat, carrots, radishes, and ginger in a bowl and set aside.

Whisk together the Nama Shoyu, raw agave nectar, lime juice, mirin, sesame oil, and chili. Pour over the papaya mixture, and toss gently. Allow to marinate for at least thirty minutes. Drain the mixture before assembling the rolls.

For the Dipping Sauce:

1 red bell pepper

1 red chili pepper, chopped with seeds

½ cup young coconut meat

2 tablespoons coconut water

Sea salt

Freshly ground black pepper to taste

Blend the bell pepper and the red chili pepper along with the coconut meat in a blender until smooth. Add coconut water as needed. Season with salt and pepper, and set aside.

For the Assembly:

1 large daikon radish or 3 medium cucumbers, peeled

½ cup finely chopped almonds

1 tablespoon almond oil

1 ripe avocado, sliced

Handful of basil leaves

Handful of raw sunflower seeds

2 tablespoons sesame seeds (black or white)

Using a sharp knife or a mandoline, cut the daikon or the cucumber into thin slices about four inches long. Use the widest slices for the assembly.

Toss the almonds with the oil, and set aside.

Lay out a sheet of daikon or cucumber, or use several overlapping slices. Place a small handful of the filling lenthwise on the slices, and top with almonds, avocado slices, basil leaves, and sprouts. Allow the leafy ends to extend beyond the ends of the wrapper. Carefully roll tightly.

Sprinkle the rolls with sesame seeds, and serve with dipping sauce.

Spring Rolls and Raw Teriyaki Sauce

(Makes 5 servings)

For the Teriyaki Sauce:

½ cup Nama Shoyu soy sauce

½ cup pure maple syrup

½ teaspoon ginger, whole

½ clove garlic

Drizzle sesame oil

Blend all the ingredients, and use as a dipping sauce.

For the Spring Rolls:

½ red bell pepper, julienned

½ large carrot, julienned

½ cup whole cilantro leaves

¼ cup fresh mint leaves, chopped

½ cup whole basil leaves

5 whole red or green cabbage leaves

Place bell pepper, carrots, cilantro, mint, and basil inside a cabbage leaf. Roll the cabbage leaf, and dip in the teriyaki sauce.

Broccoli in Hoisin Sauce with Raw Rice

(Makes 1 to 2 servings)

5 cups small broccoli florets

2 tablespoons lemon juice

3 tablespoons olive oil

1 tablespoon tamari

Mix all ingredients together until the broccoli becomes softer. Allow to marinate for about an hour.

For the Hoisin Sauce:

¼ cup tahini

1 teaspoon lemon juice

1 teaspoon yacon syrup or agave nectar

1 teaspoon apple cider vinegar

3 teaspoons tamari

½ clove garlic

½ small chili pepper, deseeded

½-centimeter-cube fresh ginger

Blend all sauce ingredients in a high-speed blender until smooth. Pour sauce over marinated broccoli, and toss well. Serve with Parsnip "Rice" (see below).

For the Parsnip "Rice":

1½ cups parsnips, peeled, chopped

1½ tablespoons pine nuts

1 tablespoon macadamia nuts

1 tablespoon light miso

1 tablespoon cold-pressed sesame oil

3 spring onions, finely chopped

Process all ingredients except the spring onions in a food processor until fluffy and rice-like. Stir in the chopped spring onions, and serve.

BREAKFASTS/DESSERTS/MISCELLANEOUS

● ●

Raw Muesli

(Makes 1 serving)

¾ cup raw nuts

About 10 dates, soaked and pitted

2 tablespoons coconut oil—optional

¼ cup fresh fruit (mango, berries, and bananas work well)

1 tablespoon fresh raw grated coconut—optional

Raw nut milk (such as almond, macadamia nut, or hemp seed milk) to taste

Using a food processor, process the nuts, dates, and coconut oil together until the nuts are almost finely ground. Combine in a bowl with fresh fruit, and top with grated coconut. Serve with nut or seed milk to taste.

● ●

Cherry Fig Cereal (Nut-Free)

(Makes 2 servings)

2 cups black mission figs, chopped

½ apple, finely diced

¼ cup ripe, chopped cherries

½ cup dried coconut ribbons or flakes

2 tablespoons Goji berries, soaked in water until soft, drained

2 tablespoons chia seeds placed in 6 tablespoons water or milk. Set aside for ten minutes.

1 teaspoon cinnamon to taste

Tiny pinch of sea salt

Other optional additions:

2 tablespoons raw cacao nibs

½ cup hemp seeds

½ cup soaked, drained raw seeds and/or chopped nuts of your choice

For the Hemp Milk:

(Makes approximately 3 cups)

¾ cup hemp seeds

3 cups water

½ cup pitted dates

1 teaspoon vanilla extract

Blend all ingredients together in a blender until smooth. Chill and serve.

• •

Lemon-Berry Ice Cream

1½ cups cashews

½ cup water

½ cup blueberries

½ cup raspberries

½ cup raw agave syrup

¼ cup lemon juice

2–3 drops lemon essential oil or lemon zest to taste—optional

Blend all ingredients in a blender until smooth and creamy. Chill the mixture in the refrigerator for at least four hours. Process the liquid through an ice cream machine according to the manufacturer's instructions.

• •

Date Bars

1 cup chopped walnuts

2 cups dates, pitted and chopped

Form chopped dates into small logs approximately two inches long by three-quarter inch thick. Roll date logs in chopped walnuts, and refrigerate for one hour.

• •

Raw Donut Holes

¾ cup almonds

¼ teaspoon sea salt

⅛ teaspoon vanilla extract

1 cup dried mango, chopped

1 cup pitted dates

6 tablespoons shredded coconut

Process almonds, salt, and vanilla in a food processor until they form a fine powder. Slowly add chopped mango and dates. Mix well. Stir in 3 tablespoons shredded coconut. To serve, use an ice cream scoop or spoon to form round balls. Roll the balls in 3 tablespoons shredded coconut.

Banana-Berry Sorbet

1 cup frozen banana in chunks

1 cup frozen mixed berries

¼ cup fresh squeezed orange juice

1 tablespoon fresh lemon or lime juice

3 tablespoons raw agave syrup

Other optional additions:

¼ cup raw granola or chopped almonds

¼ cup raw cacao nibs

You also may try different fruit combinations, such as blueberry-peach, mango-banana, pineapple-strawberry— just keep the total amount of fruit to 4 cups.

Raw Carob Energy Orbs

¾ cup nut butter (try almond or cashew but *not* peanut butter)

¼ cup tahini

½ cup sweetener (raw agave, dates, or raw honey)

1 cup sunflower seeds or sesame seeds

¼ cup of raw carob powder or cacao powder

½–¾ cup shredded coconut

Combine all ingredients, and form into balls. Refrigerate until ready to serve.

Raw Applesauce

(Makes 1½ cups)

2 apples

½ banana

½ head romaine lettuce

¼ teaspoon cinnamon

1 cup water

Process all ingredients in a food processor to desired consistency.

CPSIA information can be obtained at www.ICGtesting.com
Printed in the USA
BVOW040515030212

282098BV00001B/22/P

9 780984 896608